The Amazing Journey of Clarence Carrot

Chris Mahoney
Illustrated by LouLou Clayton

The Amazing Journey of Clarence Carrot

A New Educational Program to Promote Taste Development and Healthy Food Habits
in Young Children in a Simple, Fun, and Playful Way

Copyright © 2015 by Chris Mahoney

ALL RIGHTS RESERVED
No part of this book, covered by the copyright herein, may be reproduced, transmitted, stored, or used in any form or by any means graphic, electronic, or mechanical, including but not limited to photocopying, scanning, digitizing, taping, Web distribution, information networks, or information storage and retrieval systems, except as permitted by Section 107 or 108 of the 1976 United States Copyright Act, without the prior written permission of the author.

The content of this book is for general instruction only. Each person's physical, emotional, and spiritual condition is unique. The instruction in this book is not intended to replace or interrupt the reader's relationship with a physician or other professional. **Please consult your doctor for matters pertaining to your specific health and diet.**

Book Design: www.kameleon.media

For information or to contact the author, Chris Mahoney,
email at: **chris@chris4health.com** or visit **www.chris4health.com**

ISBN 978-0-692-39061-0

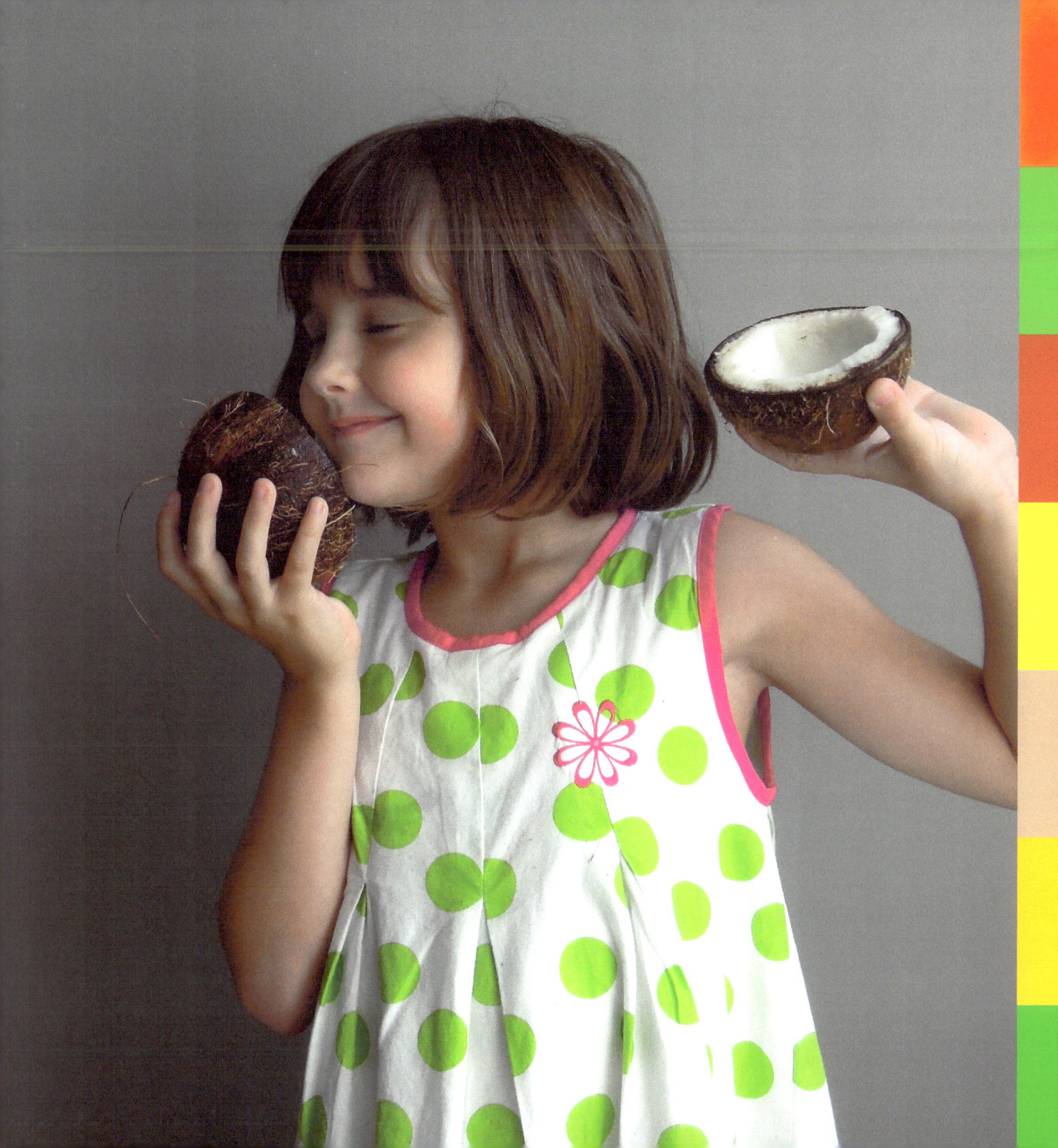

Table of Contents

9	Dedication
9	Introduction
10	My Story

CHAPTER ONE
12	**Taste and Healthy Eating**
14	Encourage Taste Development
16	Focus on Young Children

CHAPTER TWO
18	**Getting Parents Involved in This Amazing Journey**
21	In Every Child Lurks a 'Taste Champion'...!
22	Nutrition and Moving

CHAPTER THREE
24	**Have Great Taste Fun!**
27	How Does Clarence Carrot's Program Work?
29	5 Helpful Strategies Used in All Activities

CHAPTER FOUR
30	**Meet Clarence Carrot, "The Taste Champion", and his friends**
42	Tom Tomato's Birthday Party

CHAPTER FIVE
46	**Introduce the Five Senses**
48	Activity 1: A Sensory Stroll
49	Activity 2: Make a Book
49	Activity 3: Who is Who??
49	Activity 4: Tasting for Beginners

CHAPTER SIX

50   **The Amazing Journey**
54   Activity 1: Photo Friend
55   Activity 2: Let's Make a Little 'Elf' Poem
56   Activity 3: Puzzle Game
56   Activity 4: Play Copy Cat
56   Activity 5: Magnifying Glass
56   Activity 6: Traffic Light
56   Activity 7: Explore Colors

CHAPTER SEVEN

58   **The Little Honey Bread**
64   Activity 1: Explore the Instruments
65   Activity 2: Tell the Honey Bread Story Again
65   Activity 3: Move and Play
65   Activity 4: Bake and Taste
66   Activity 5: Snaps, Crackles, Pops, and Crunches
67   Activity 6: Listen and Dance to the Song

CHAPTER EIGHT

68   **Fun at the Farm**
72   The Touch Box
72   Activity 1: Search for the Carrot
72   Activity 2: Choose and Touch
72   Activity 3: Guess What I'm Feeling
73   Activity 4: Little Chefs
73   Activity 5: Chop, Slice and TASTE!

CHAPTER NINE

74   **Mia Bella and the Little Cloud**

80	Activity 1: Tasting Without Smelling
80	Activity 2: The Nose Knows Matching Game
81	Activity 3: Smell Boxes

CHAPTER TEN

82	**Meeting Sisters Sweet, Salty, Sour, and Bitter**
87	Activity 1: Identify the Four Basic Tastes: Sweet, Salty, Sour, and Bitter
88	Activity 2: Can You Recognize Sweet, Salty, Sour, and Bitter in a Variety of Foods?
88	Activity 3: Salted Water
89	Activity 4: SWEET Tooth

CHAPTER ELEVEN

90	**Finale: An Unforgettable Taste Festival**
92	Activity 1: A Fruity Atmosphere
92	Activity 2: A Medal for the "Taste Champions"
92	Activity 3: Young Chefs
92	Activity 4: Cheers!
92	Activity 5: Let's Move!
93	Activity 6: Dance to the Music!

THE SUITCASE

96	All Materials Needed for the Program
97	The Taste Pass
98	Acknowledgements
99	Resources

Dedication

To all the children in my life who love to listen to stories with curiosity and wonder. May all the stories and activities in this book make them real "Taste Champions"!

> DO NOT GROW OLD
> NO MATTER HOW LONG YOU LIVE.
> NEVER CEASE TO STAND LIKE CURIOUS CHILDREN
> BEFORE THE GREAT MYSTERY INTO WHICH WE WERE BORN.
>
> Albert Einstein

Introduction

Clarence Carrot invites children on an Amazing Journey - with stories and activities that challenge everybody to become a "Taste Champion"!

Children are encouraged to look at food differently: with curiosity and wonder - opening their minds towards unknown deliciousness while learning how to keep their bodies healthy. Adults and children will enjoy traveling with Clarence to a world of new scents, colors, flavors, and lots of fun!

Stories and "Do and Think" activities focus on observing food and learning about nutrition. All 5 senses are used to explore and discover new, yummy things to eat. Through listening, playing, talking, crafting, making music, moving, smelling, and tasting, kids will absorb information to promote good health for their entire lives!

So, come along! Join Clarence Carrot on his Amazing Journey and get inspired to help children become "**Taste Champions**"!

Chris Mahoney - chris4health

My Story

Looking back at my life, I see where my love of healthy food originated and how it became a gift for myself and others, culminating in my exciting food project for children.

Child number eight in a family of 10, I was born in Gent, Belgium. Living in a house bustling with family, friends, and neighbors, was challenging, especially escaping the noise and controlling eyes of the elder ones. Fortunately, I went to school at a young age with Andre, my older brother by two years who was also my best friend.

After school we stayed outside as much as possible. My father's huge garden was our playground. Hide and seek games were enjoyed in several places of earthy, delicious scents: the vegetable area, the patch with berries and fruit trees, or the flower garden with my dad's bee cases. In the back, under the hazel tree was a shed with large barrels of apples, fermenting into cider. We spent hours picking string beans, tomatoes, berries, cherries, apples, pears... We helped harvest the honey which smelled and tasted like local flowers and herbs.

Picking flowers and bringing them home for my very active mom was one of my favorite activities. A local politician and women's rights activist, she also worked as an accountant in the city. But most importantly, she was the household coordinator. Everybody had to take care of everybody. Even as a young child, I loved helping in the kitchen! (My mom was also a great bedtime storyteller, and I feel fortunate to have had such a role model.)

I enjoyed a fun and adventurous adolescence and decided to become a teacher. I loved the atmosphere and my courses in college. Upon graduating, I taught at the Practice School for Teachers in my home town Sint-Amandsberg. I had a class of my own (6th graders), and also mentored teachers-to-be and gave model classes. My students and mentees were happy to have a "young," enthusiastic teacher. It was very interesting! I had access to the newest learning methods and tools, and several topics kept my mind focused on research.

Practicing "Active Listening," after Thomas Gordon's Teacher Effectiveness Training, helped me to work on a high quality relationship with my students and their parents. I became more aware of the power of telling stories and "learning through play" - helping children understand and share their world while being active, exploring... and most importantly: having fun!

At 21, I married, and by 26, we had two children: Sam, our oldest, and Liesbeth. Positive mothering and having a happy family was, and still is, the goal of my life. While teaching, I managed to take cooking classes with top Belgium chefs to spoil my beloved ones with good food. The meals gave great pleasure to us all.

Later, after becoming single again, I studied intercultural diversity. I learned about the struggles of Turkish and Moroccan immigrants seeking a better life in Belgium, about racism and discrimination, human rights, and equal opportunities. I've shared this knowledge with my own children as well as my students.

After 27 years working with children in schools, it was time for a change. I started a job as an educational expert for the Flemish government on projects to raise awareness of intercultural diversity, the globalization movement, and equal opportunities. I worked with thoughtful, caring and creative people.

Since the "New Belgians" came from all over the planet, I experimented with recipes and had the good fortune to taste the "World Kitchen."

Sam started to travel all over the world, combining his job as IT specialist and his passion for sports triathlons. Liesbeth married and moved to the USA. She introduced me to Dennis, the kindest, most generous man I have ever met. After my last project, a traveling exhibition about "the power of enterprising women in developing countries," I moved to Pennsylvania and married him.

My stories about a carrot entertained my granddaughters, Paulien and Molly, while we sat at the kitchen table finishing our plates. The idea of creating a tool for educators, to make parents aware of taste development in children, grew day by day. After a while, the project of encouraging children to become "Taste Champions" was real. Graduating in 2013 as a Holistic Health Coach at the Institute for Integrative Nutrition has given me significant knowledge, expertise and support to launch my tool.

The title of my book is, The Amazing Journey of Clarence Carrot, and I can tell you, Clarence and I have a lot in common. I'm pretty sure you will love him!

CHAPTER ONE

Taste and Healthy Eating

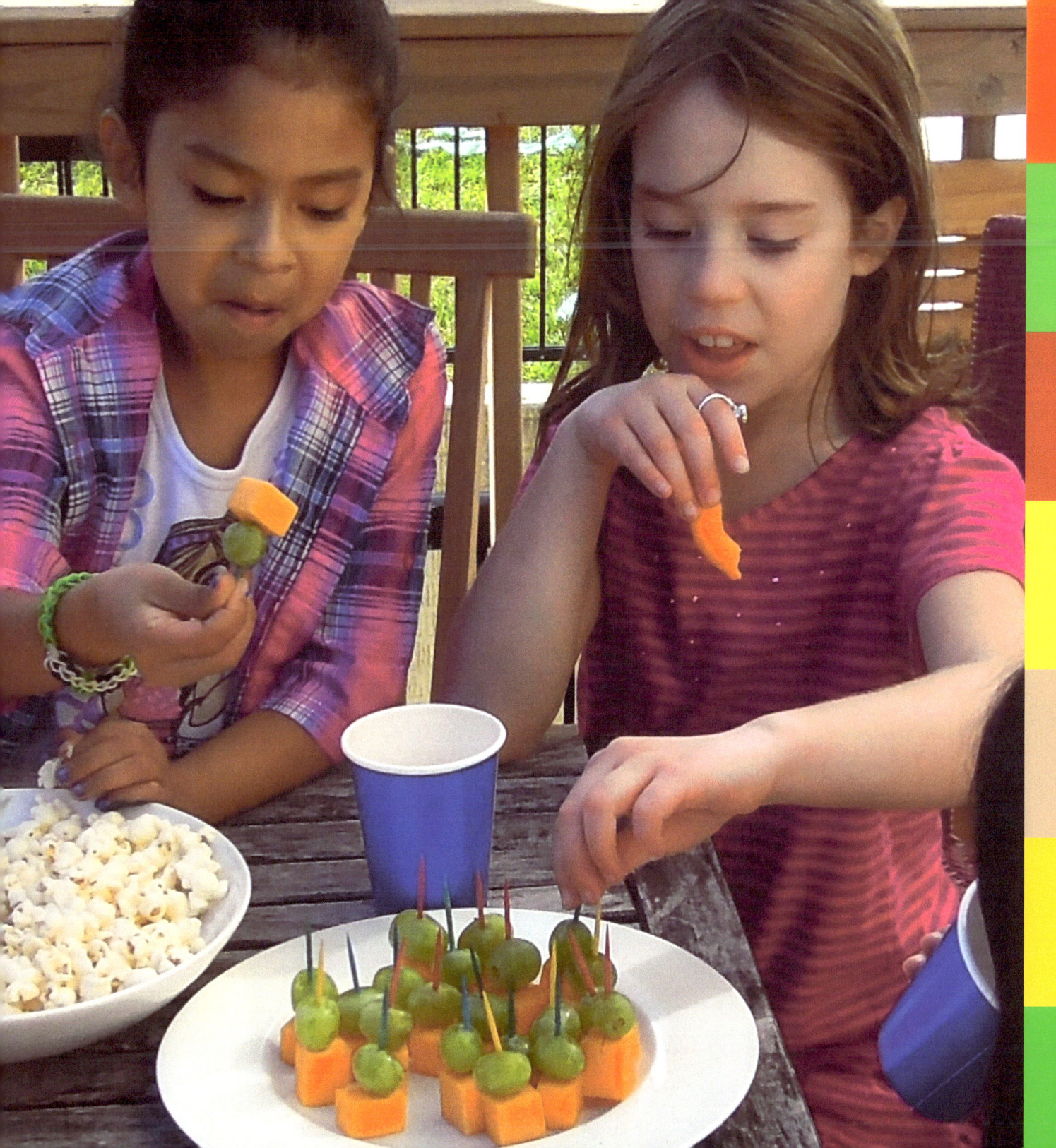

For children, taste is the beginning of enjoying food and the foundation of a healthy eating pattern. The development of the sense of taste in young children is an important way to help them eat a variety of healthy foods.

The shaping of taste preferences begins in the womb and continues throughout the rest of our lives. For newborns, the taste sense is the most important and most developed of all senses.

Evolution most likely dictated the sensible preference for sweetness. It can be explained by the fact that a sweet taste indicates a source of energy (carbohydrates), which is non-poisonous, and thus safe to eat. A bitter taste, in turn, warns us of toxic foods. Similar evolutionary programming is assumed for other tastes: an acidic taste may warn against spoiled food, whereas a salty taste may hint at minerals. The taste quality "umami" (savory) indicates a good protein source as it naturally occurs in animal foods.

Children often like foods they have eaten in pleasant situations and reject dishes linked to something negative. Tasty foods (high energy density, high fat and sugar content; e.g., desserts), are commonly served on pleasant occasions such as celebrations or when guests visit. In contrast, foods considered less tasty (e.g. vegetables), are often consumed under pressure: "Eat your veggies or you won't get any dessert." This double-negative coupling increases the popularity of energy-dense, tasty dishes and the aversion against less savory foods.

The body is like a "house" that has to be constructed and maintained. Children need a lot of building materials, essential for development of their bones, muscles, and organs. They are also used for daily activities, such as walking, talking, breathing, playing, learning… Research shows that children who eat breakfast perform better academically. Did you know that 20% of children do not eat breakfast every day?

A healthy diet helps prevent conditions such as tooth decay, obesity, and diarrhea. An unhealthy diet can weaken the immune system and leave children vulnerable to illness. Adults with unhealthy eating behaviors have a higher risk of high blood pressure, heart disease, cancer, and diabetes. Because we want our children to become healthy and happy adults, we have to invest time in teaching them healthy eating patterns at a very young age.

Encourage Taste Development

To ensure that children eat healthy foods, it is important to influence their food preferences. The greater the variety of fruits and vegetables that they like, the more diverse their eating pattern will become. Children's food preferences change as they grow older, mostly under the influence of their environment. If encouraged, young children will discover new flavors and broaden their diets.

This is not an easy process for every child. Therefore, we must stimulate them to develop their sense of taste as much as possible. Said above Children are born with a "sweet tooth," and they have difficulty with sour and bitter flavors. Many kids are naturally suspicious of unfamiliar foods. They may quickly categorize them as "yummy" or "yucky" - sometimes before the foods have passed their lips.

"Good tasters" are not afraid to taste something they do not like. They see it as part of the adventure. Without tasting a few disgusting mouthfuls, they would not know how to tell when something tastes amazing.

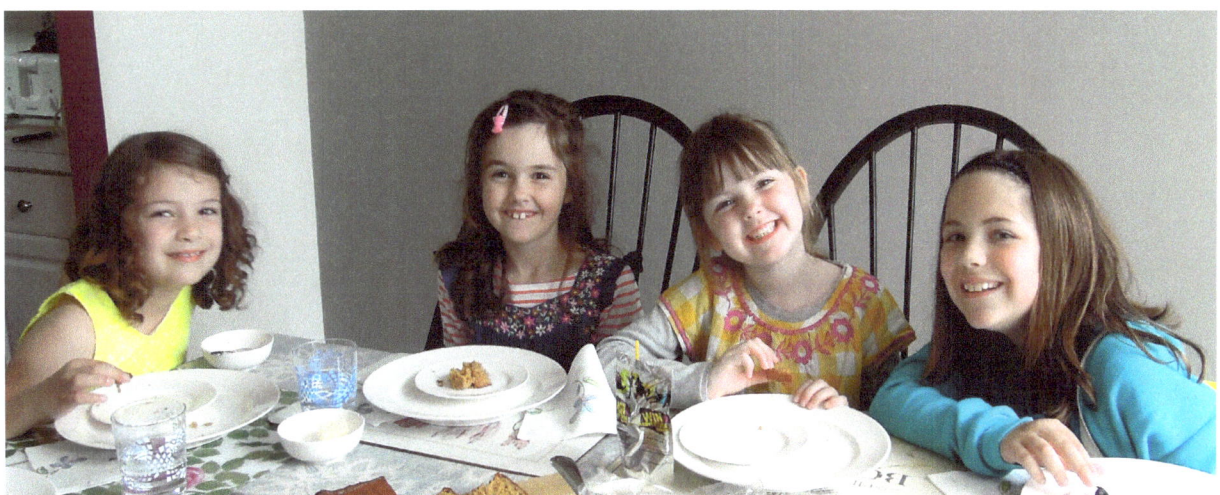

The Amazing Journey of Clarence Carrot

Focus on Young Children

Young children depend on their families, caregivers and teachers, to support their well-being and to promote positive development, including eating behaviors. Children's food preferences and willingness to try new foods are influenced by the people around them. The development of eating behaviors is a dynamic process that begins in infancy and continues throughout life.

It is shocking, but research shows that toddlers are eating in an unhealthy manner. Only one in five eat sufficient vegetables, and half drink too many sugared beverages. More and more children struggle with weight issues. This is a worrying national trend.

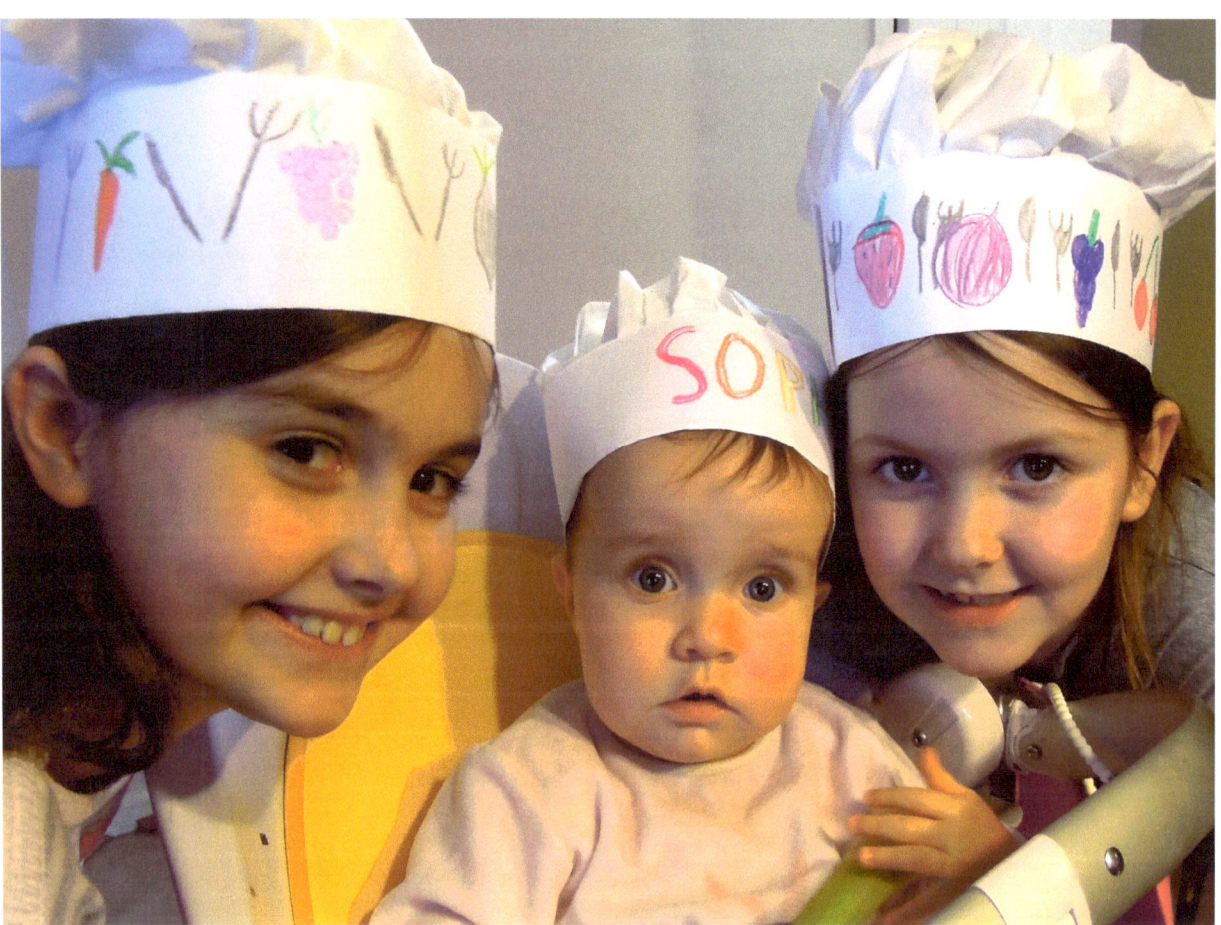

Genetics and the contexts in which foods are presented are two key factors that underpin the development of eating behaviors. Although parents provide a child's biological predisposition, which may affect factors like taste perception, they are not the only adults influencing the development of a child's eating behaviors. Every family member or caregiver interacting with a child at meals or snacks has the potential to do so.

In center- and home-based child-care settings and schools, family, teachers and child-care provider influence children's eating behaviors by the foods they offer, the behaviors they model, and their social interactions with children at snack and mealtimes.

The following are a few examples of how these factors influence eating behaviors. Repeated exposure to a new food reduces a child's fear of the food and helps increase acceptance. (Although experiments vary, researchers tell us that offering a food 10 to 15 times, appears necessary to increase a child's food acceptance.).

Observing adults eating and enjoying a variety of foods makes these foods more appealing to children. (If adults are eating high-fat, calorie-dense foods, children will follow their lead). In contrast, children who are pressured to eat specific foods learn to dislike them, and restricted access to some foods, such as cookies or potato chips, often results in overconsumption of those foods when children are free to make their own food choices.

Most children naturally demonstrate fears of new foods. Neophobia - or fear of "the new" - is a protective behavior observed in omnivores, including humans, that helps prevent consumption of harmful substances. We can decrease children's fears by creating supportive environments with enjoyable, nutritious, and fun early-food experiences.

Children and their parents deserve special attention in the process of "taste education." It has been shown that the context in which family meals take place has an important role in shaping eating behavior. Preferences and aversions are highly individual, but may display clear familial and social links.

Since taste preferences are stable and may last a lifetime, special care should be dedicated to the meal setting. Negative influences such as arguments during meals should be avoided. Leaving children some room for their food choices and showing certain calmness towards temporary food aversions can be key in the development of taste preferences.

CHAPTER TWO

Getting Parents Involved in This Amazing Journey

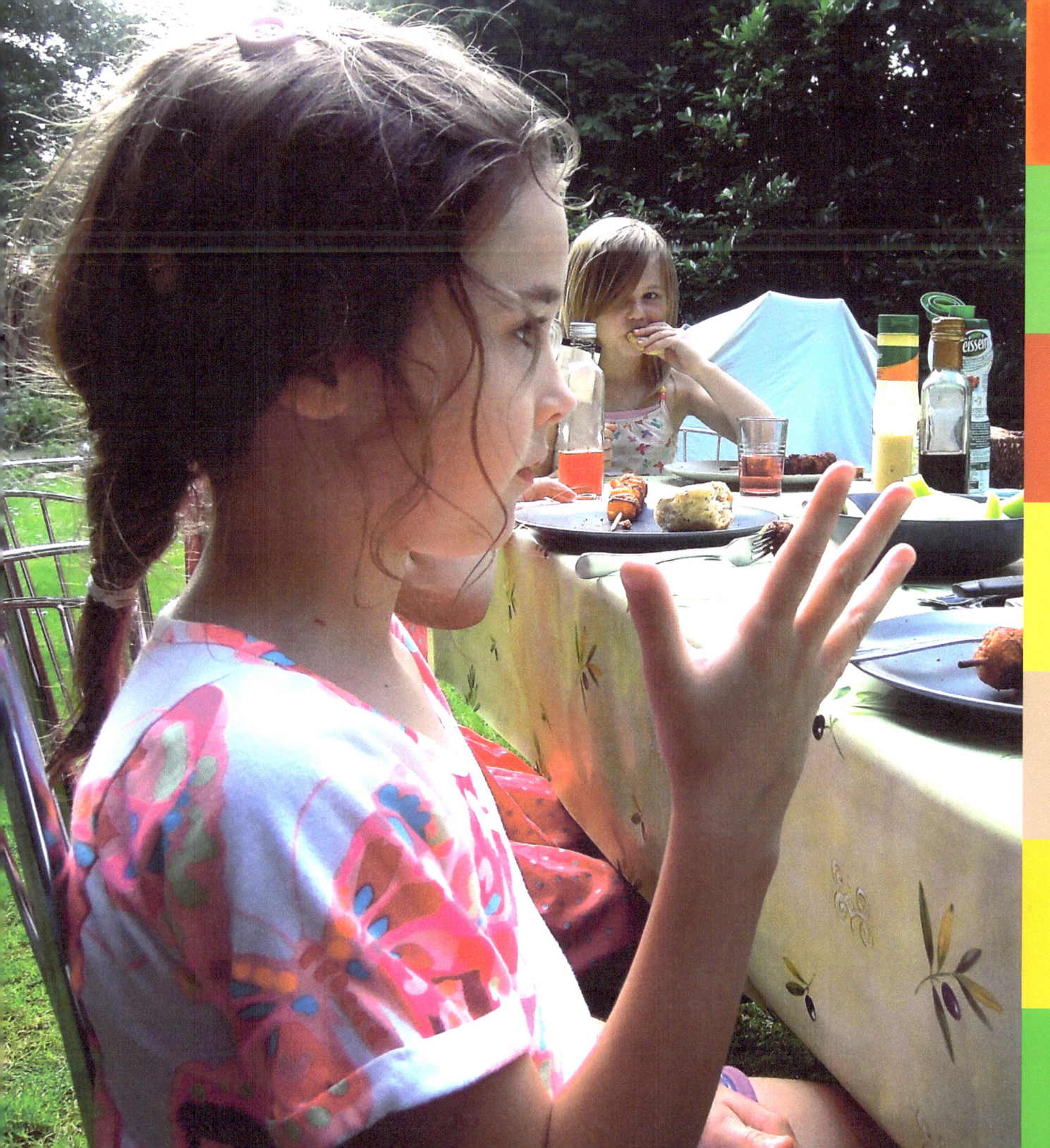

The Amazing Journey of Clarence Carrot

Before you begin the program, invite parents to review it. Show them Clarence Carrot and his friends, and explain the importance of taste development. The goal of making their child a "Taste Champion" will trigger parents to co-operate, and in many cases there will be "life style changes" in their own eating habits. Educating parents through their children is a double win!

The activities in this book expose children to foods from different cultures and provide opportunities to learn more about their friends. The acceptance of new foods is a slow process. Particularly for ages 2 to 5, persistence is essential.

A parent/teacher/caregiver may think it is best to hold off on introducing food variety until a child's fearful responses decrease. Instead, it is important to offer positive exposure to an assortment of foods throughout early childhood. Although children are skeptical of many foods during these early years, the diversity of foods they accept is greater in this developmental phase than in later childhood.

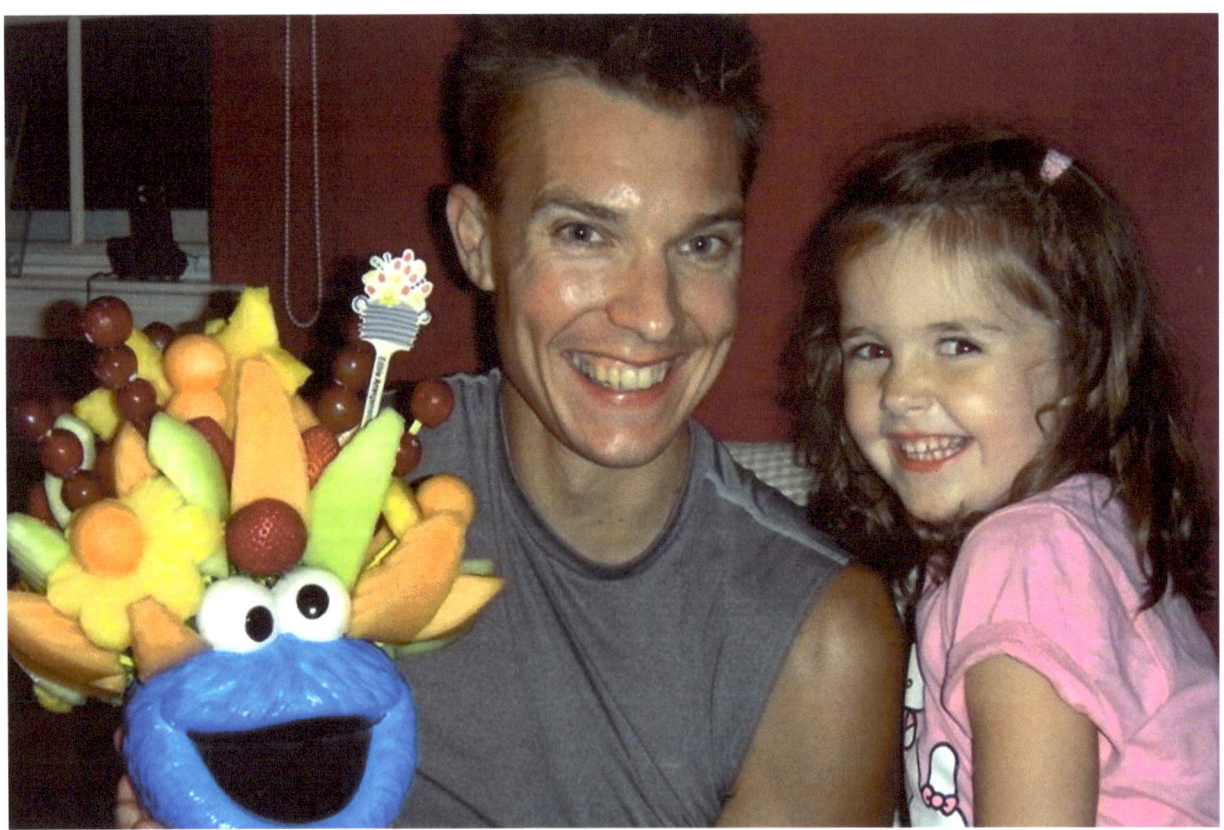

In Every Child Lurks a 'Taste Champion' ... !

A lot of children struggle with string beans, broccoli, or other veggies and fruits. Fries, pizza, and chocolate are big favorites!

Today, children live in an environment where fast food is everywhere, often for little money and large portions. The food industry spends massive amounts of money on advertising to make unhealthy food attractive! Young children are especially responsive to these messages because they have a natural preference for sweet and salty flavors.

"I don't like this!" often makes mealtime in a lot of families a daily battleground.

By using the program, The Amazing Journey of Clarence Carrot, you will organize simple, creative taste-moments with variety in color, texture, and taste, to appeal to young children. When serving a new item such as a cucumber or apple in one of the activities, you will encourage children to look, smell, touch, and taste the (new) food. It is perfectly acceptable for a child to avoid a new vegetable the first several times it is offered. Inviting children to touch and smell the food helps them take small steps toward tasting.

Encouraging, rather than requiring, children to eat a food is the key objective. Clarence Carrot, the "Taste Champion", teaches young kids to enjoy tastes and supports parents to help their children learn to eat well.

At the end of the program you will have the opportunity to host a (classroom) party with all of the foods and to invite parents to enjoy the event with their children. Parents will be delighted to watch their kids role-playing the stories, serving healthy snacks, and best of all, see the happy face of their child wearing the medal of a "Taste Champion."

Nutrition and Moving

Young children need healthy nutrition and physical activity in order to grow, learn, and succeed, both in school and in life. However, early childhood obesity is a barrier to their growth and development.

Being physically active improves children's overall health. When they move, kids just feel good. Physical activity helps children stay at a healthy weight and promotes strength, flexibility and endurance. Moving also enhances their motor skills, social skills, and brain development, develops and maintains strong bones, fosters better sleep, and most importantly, builds confidence about themselves and their bodies as they grow.

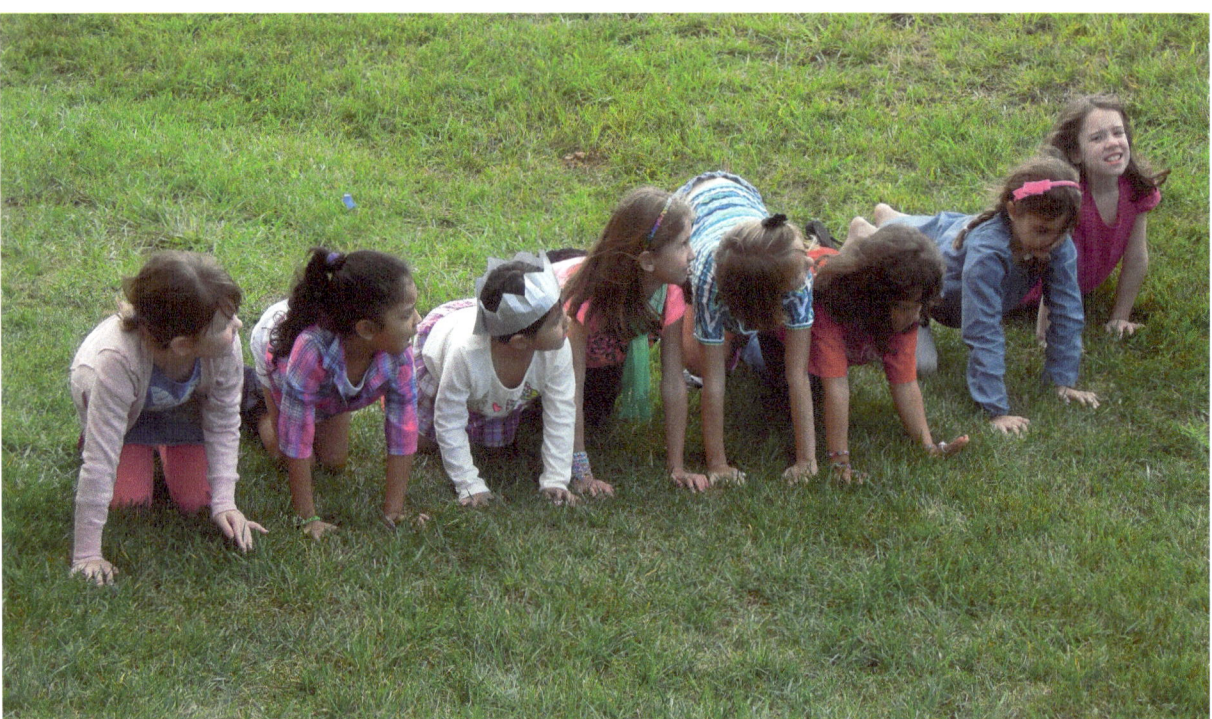

Since many children are in childcare or school throughout the week, it's important to give youngsters of all ages daily opportunities to be physically active in a safe play space, surrounded by positive and responsive grown-ups like yourself. Despite massive attention to healthy diet and exercise, there are still prejudices and misconceptions about healthy eating and exercise.

Think of the word "light" or "lean" on product packaging; one gets a false impression that the product is guaranteed to be healthy. Unfortunately, the food industry advertises and sells a wide range of products with a "healthy" look, which don't deliver health benefits. This makes it difficult for parents to make the best choices.

The Amazing Journey of Clarence Carrot helps sort out the confusion. The program offers parents, teachers and caregivers, easy-to-understand information on nutrition, as well as developmentally appropriate physical activities for every story in this book!

Clarence Carrot, the Taste Champion encourages eating healthy food and moving!

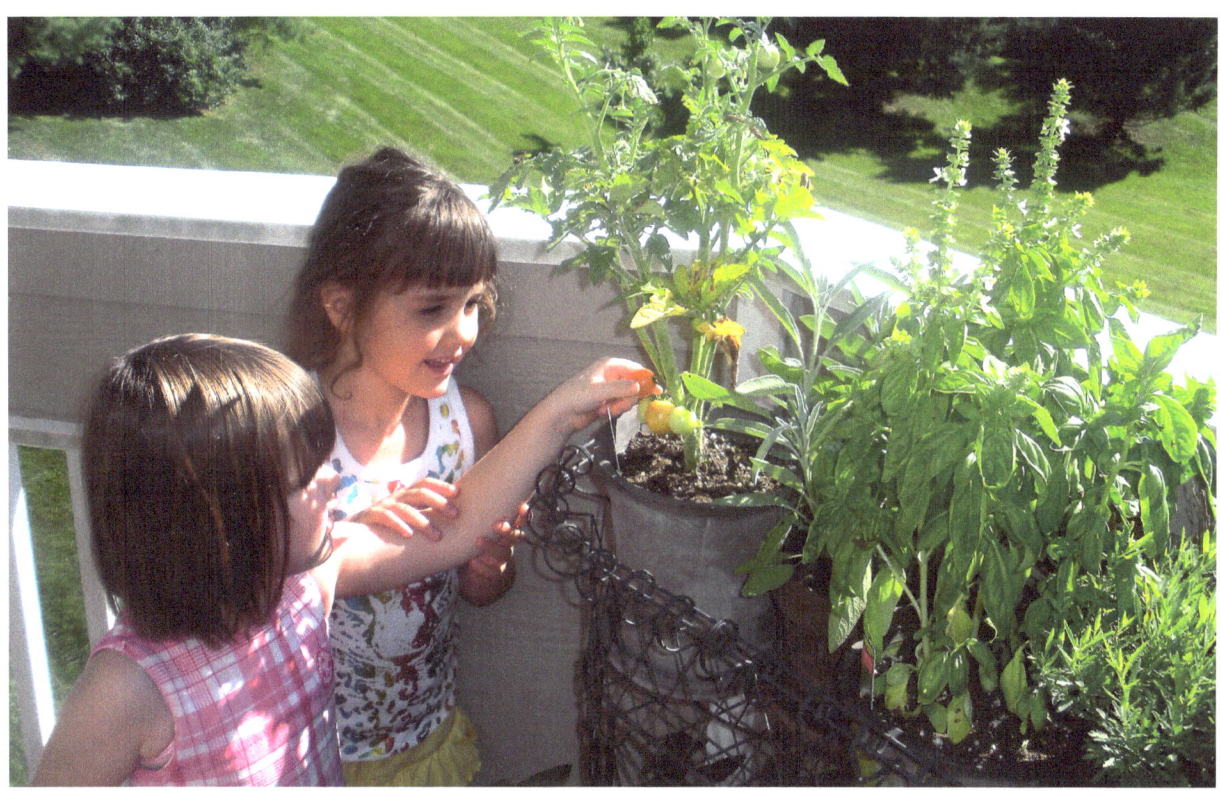

CHAPTER THREE

Have Great Taste Fun!

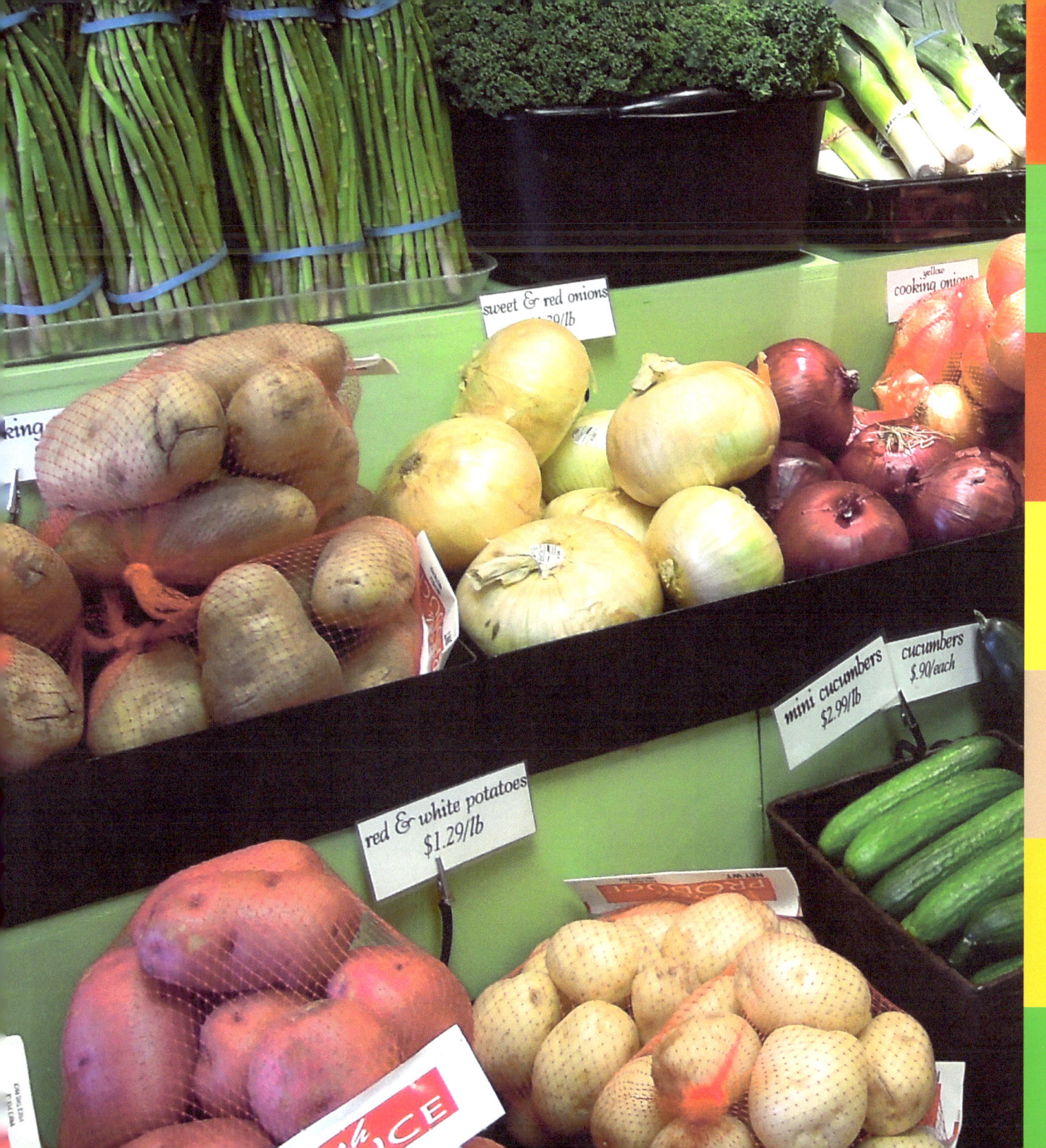

The Amazing Journey of Clarence Carrot turns food experimentation into a game instead of an obligation. When "playing," kids are more likely to try new things. They may discover there is a lot more to mealtime than just peanut butter and jelly!

Because children are different, this program offers a variety of stories, games, and activities to introduce them to new healthy foods, reinforced by sensory exploration.

Sufficient directions allow you to independently get started. Children will join an amazing journey through the world of our 5 senses: feeling, tasting, smelling, hearing, and looking, as they play, experiment, learn, and most of all... have fun!! Without effort they will experiment with the four basic tastes: sour, salty, sweet, and bitter.

Children must learn to taste, just as they learned to take their first steps by falling and getting back up. They also learn to appreciate flavors by tasting foods and spitting out things they do not like. Learning to taste does not work by itself. It certainly is worth the trouble to help children with this process. The more flavors they like, the healthier they will eat.

Teaching children about the five senses is a good way to help them understand their bodies. Likewise, it increases self esteem, because they are discovering new and exciting things about themselves.

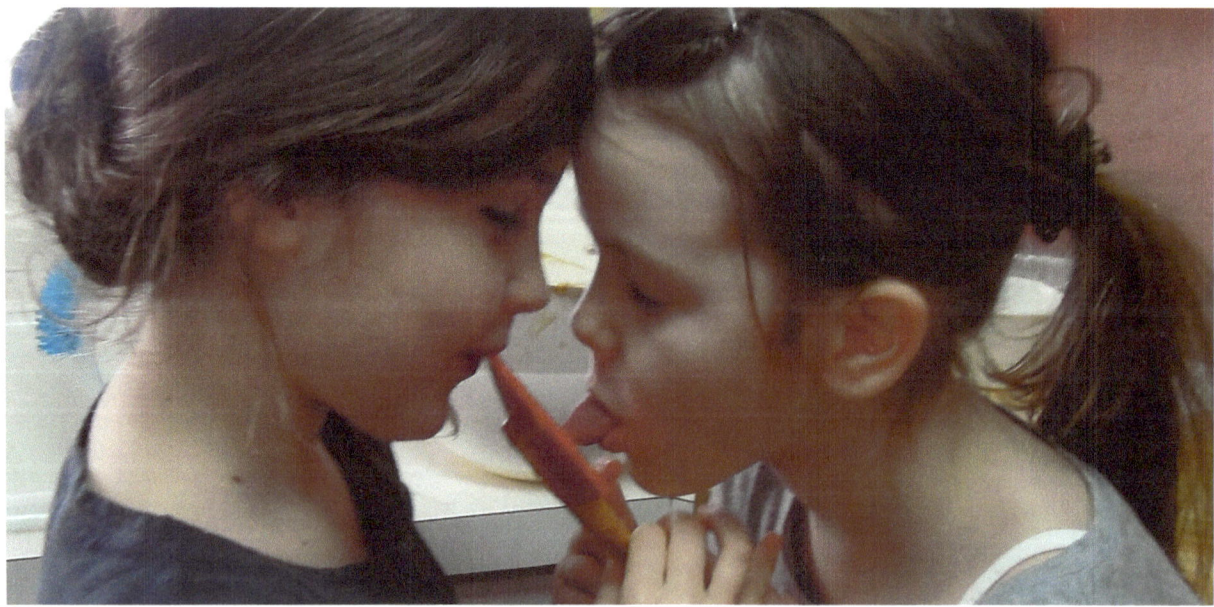

How Does Clarence Carrot's Program Work?

Children listen to stories about Clarence Carrot, and he encourages them to participate in activities to become "Taste Champions" just like him. All is supported with a suitcase (tool box) filled with pictures and materials that you will need. You can find the entire list at the end of this book. There are five stories, followed by a bunch of activities - each focusing on one of the five senses.

Have fun! Tell the stories in a highly dramatic way to increase the children's interest in the program. Also, it's very important to let them interact while you are sharing the stories.

Depending on the time available and the space, you can choose which activities to offer and develop your own project.

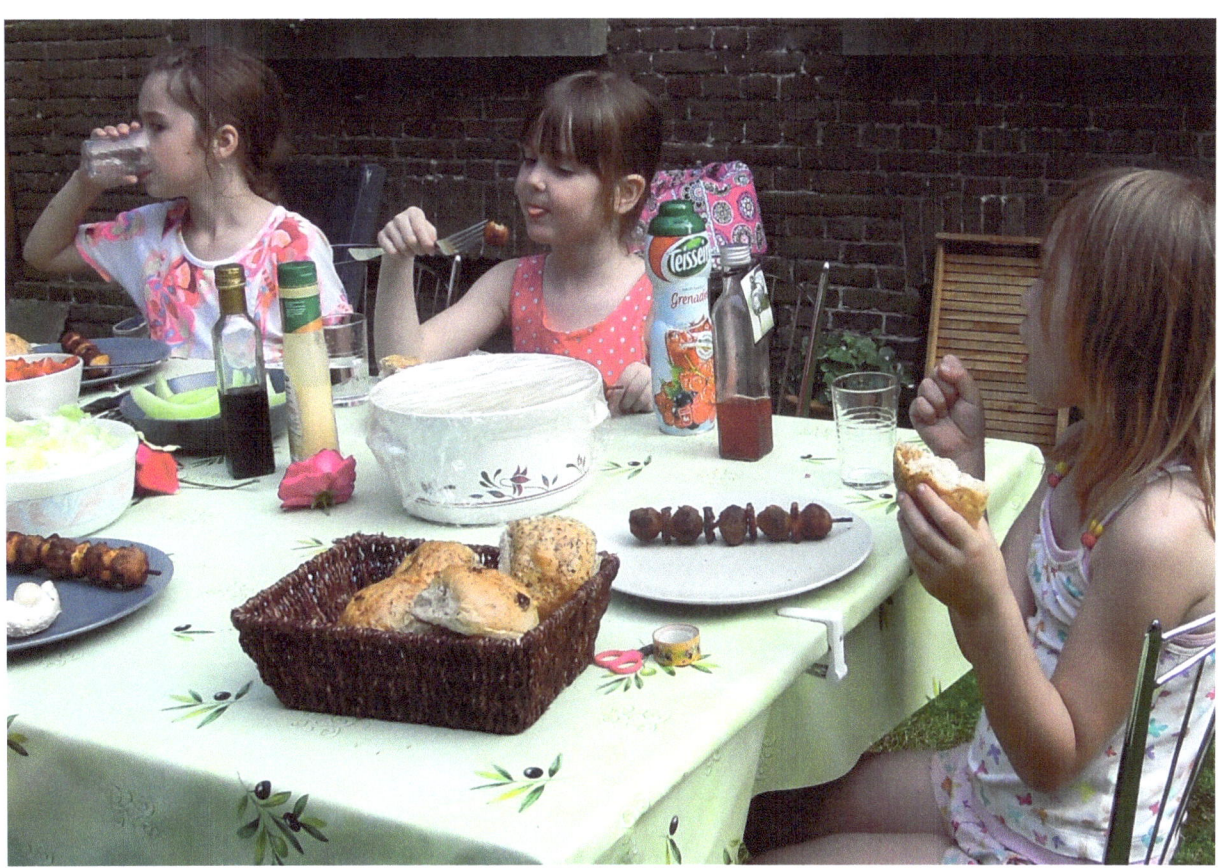

As you know, a five-year-old does not have the same capabilities as a child of eight. Therefore, it is important to differentiate activities according to the age of the children.

Since these activities offer children the opportunity to look, hear, feel, smell, and taste different foods, you may take that literally. This means you will need a number of ingredients.

Initially, you can buy them yourself. (Since the portions are tidbits, it should not mean a significant layout of funds.) Later, why not include the children so they can get an idea of the variety of vegetables, fruits, and other healthy products available. This could include an excursion to a farmers market, a produce place, or a grocery store in the neighborhood.

When you go with the children to the store, you will soon learn that there are many veggies and fruit varieties they do not know.

And most importantly: involve parents in the whole taste project!

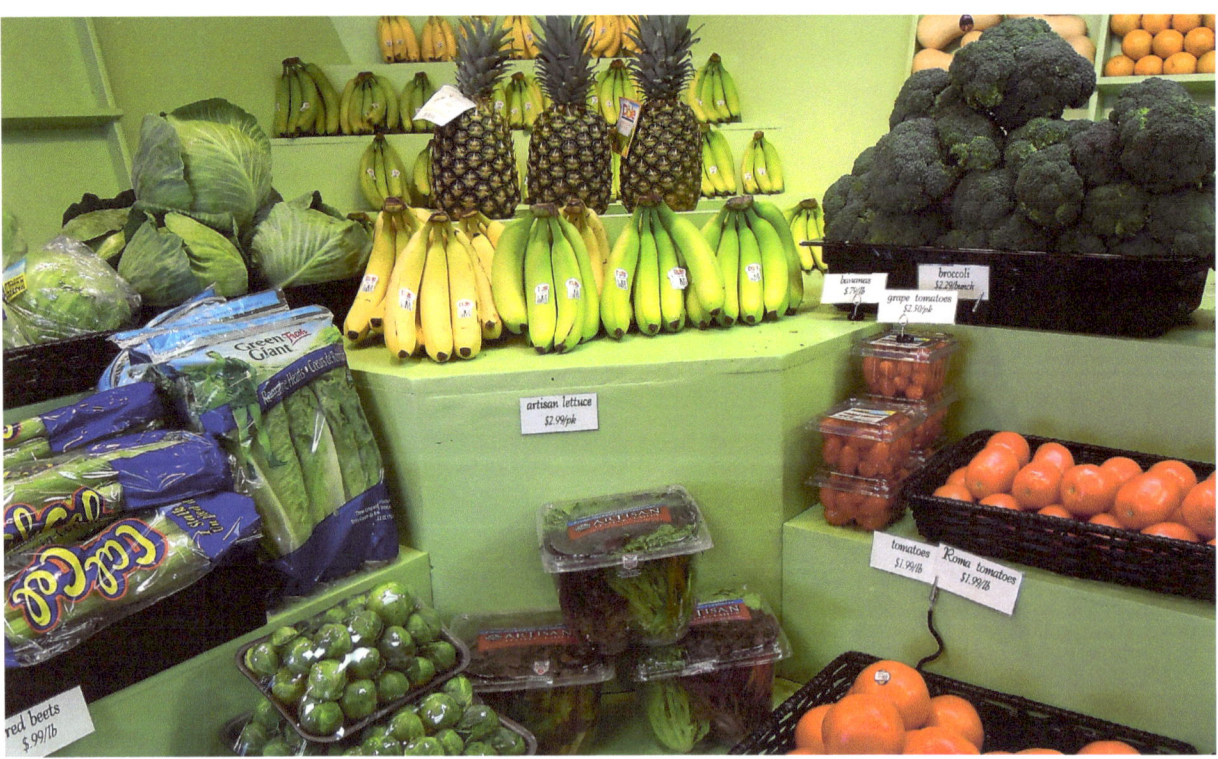

5 Helpful Strategies Used in All Activities

Recognize and Name
Here is a great opportunity to introduce lots of veggies and fruits that children do not know. Teach children the names of these new foods, and in fun ways, test their recall.

Describe
Produce has specific colors, shapes, structures... Encourage children to touch and describe everything.

Watch, Hear, Taste, Smell, Touch
Allow children to feel "safe to taste." Explain that when tasting food, we use different senses and that "tasting" does not mean "eating." Inform them that a little piece of food is enough for tasting, and they can spit it out if they do not like it.

Know the Four Different Tastes: Sweet, Sour, Bitter, Salty
Help children identify the different tastes.

What Is Yummy and What Is Not?
Encourage the children to say what they like and what they do not like. Ask them why. Is it because of its taste? Its look? Its smell? Lots of children do not like what they do not 'know' or what they have never tasted. Allow children to talk freely.

CHAPTER FOUR

Meet Clarence Carrot,
"The Taste Champion", and his friends

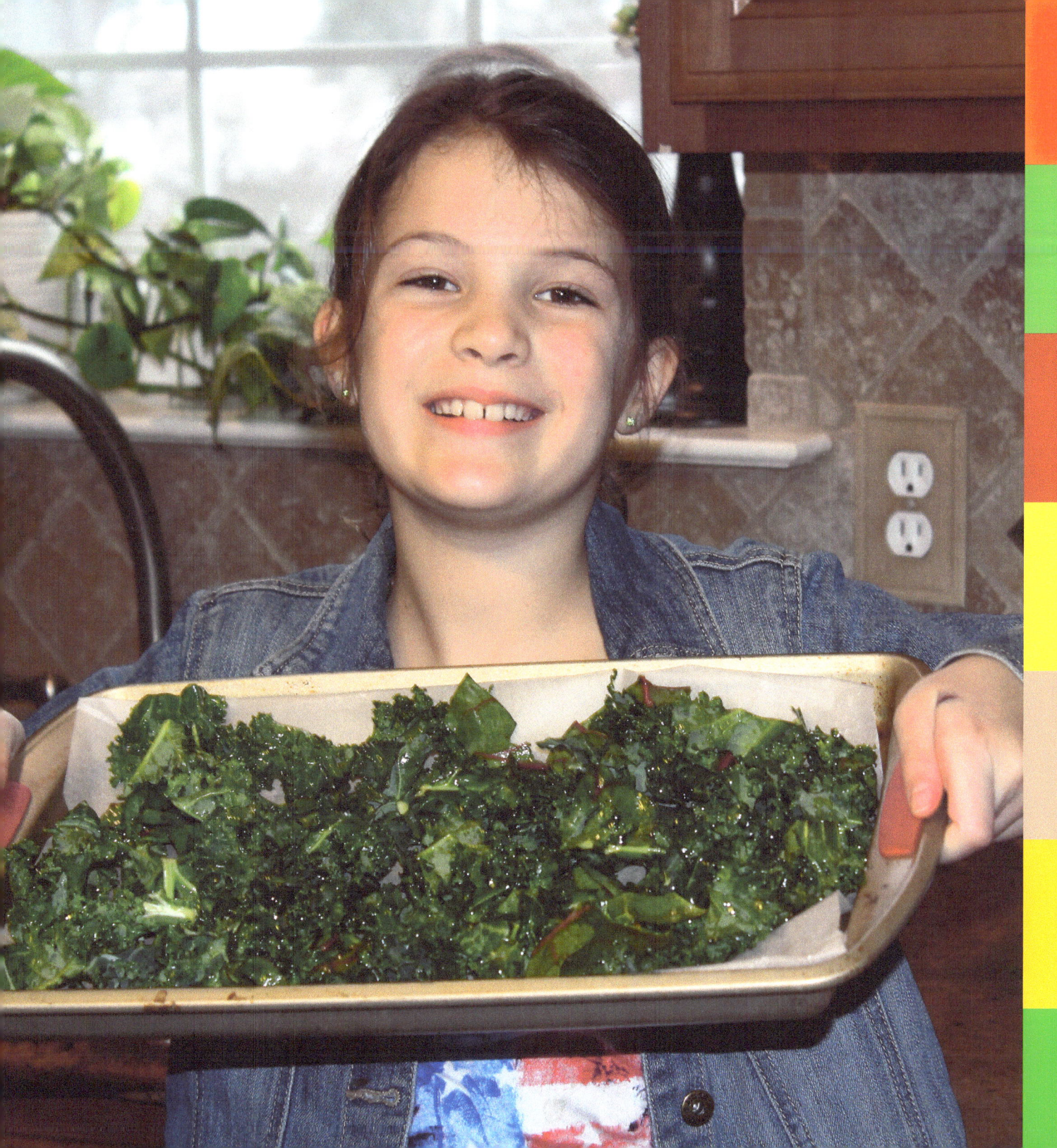

Goals of the Chapter
> Children "meet" fruit and vegetables and name them correctly.
> Children understand the story, and they answer direct questions.
> Children can organize a series of pictures, and they are able to reconstruct the story with them.
> Children understand the message of the program.
> Children are eager to taste.

Time
30-40 minutes

Materials
> Suitcase with Clarence Carrot in a basket
> Pictures of the 8 characters
> Pictures of an apple, cheese, a strawberry, a banana, cauliflower and a lemon (you can also show 'real' food!)

Setting
Children are sitting in a circle.

Directions for the narrator:
Act out the story as if it really happened! Use the pictures while telling the story. Let the children spontaneously interact.

One day I heard somebody knocking at my door.

KNOCK, KNOCK, KNOCK!

I opened it, and I saw two little eyes and a big smile... an orange creature.

**"There you are, finally!
I'm so happy that I found you,"** it said.

Is that a vegetable sitting on a huge suitcase?

"Do I know you?" I asked.

"Let me introduce myself: I am Clarence Carrot," he said.

Then he started a whole story about a vegetable garden in Belgium, far away across the ocean in Europe.

The carrot had run away from the garden and started a long trip all around the world... to find us!

Then he said, "I've brought a suitcase full of fun "things" and a book full of stories and pictures."

Would you like to meet him? Come, let's call him:
CLARENCE CARROT!

He is smart, right to the point, and he wants you to know his friends, too!

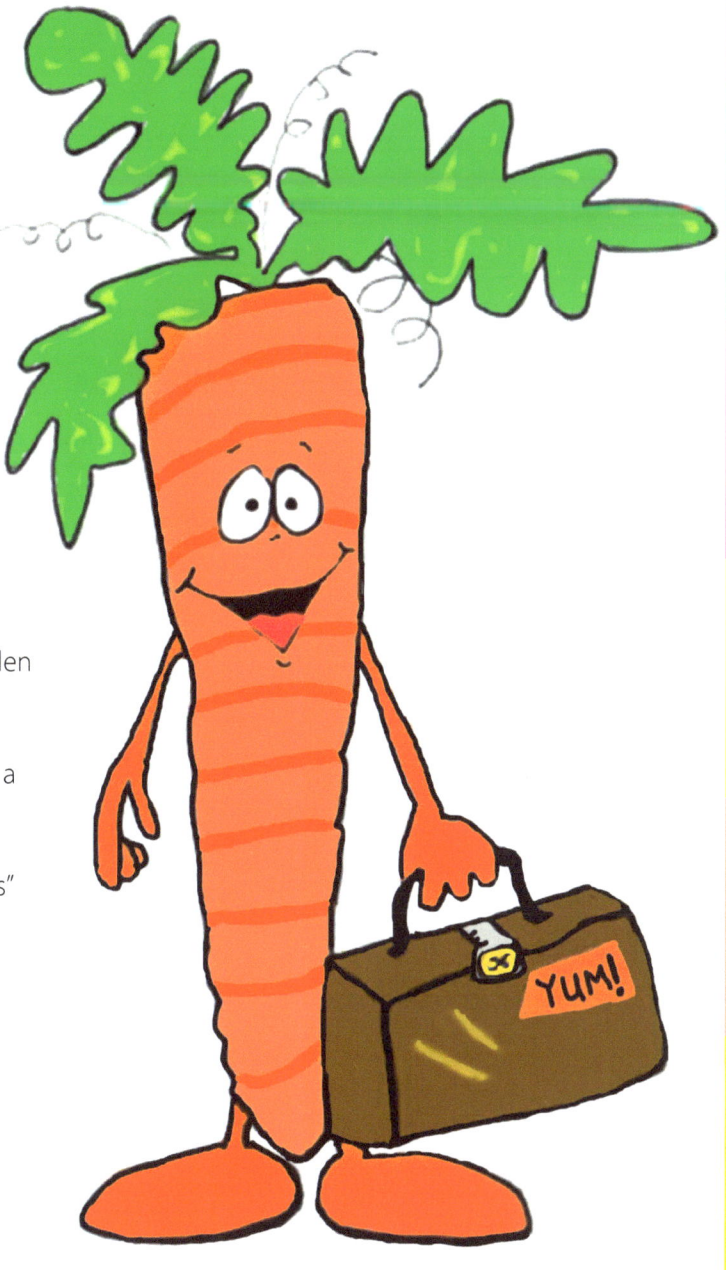

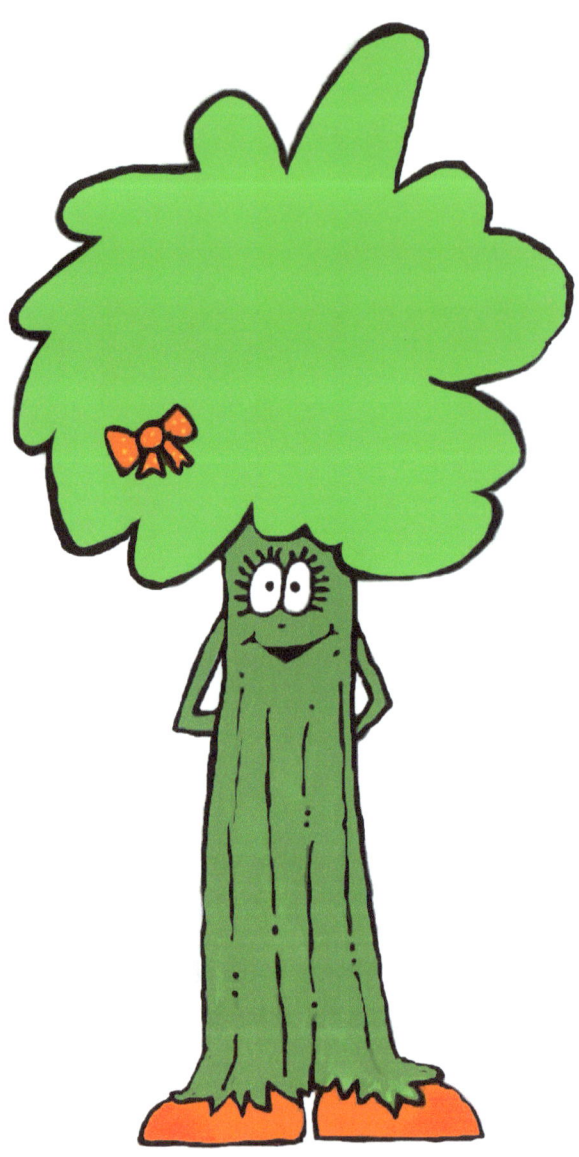

Let's start with...**Bonnie Broccoli!**
She is full of health and always ready to help.

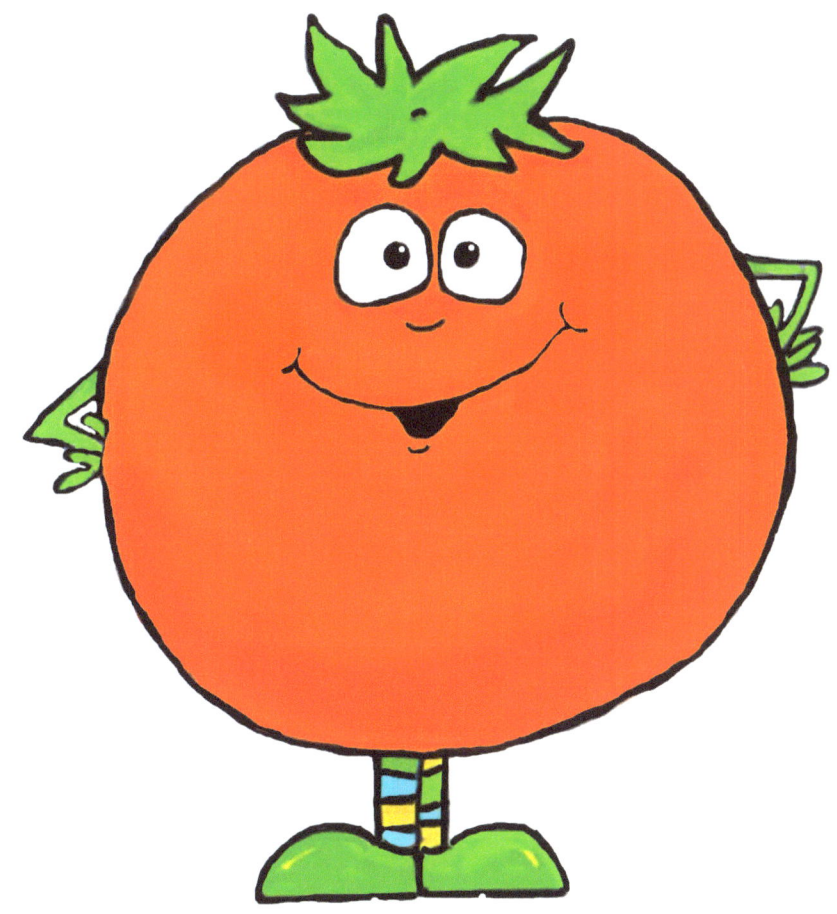

And here comes...**Tom Tomato**!
He has a round belly and he likes to salsa dance.

The Amazing Journey of Clarence Carrot

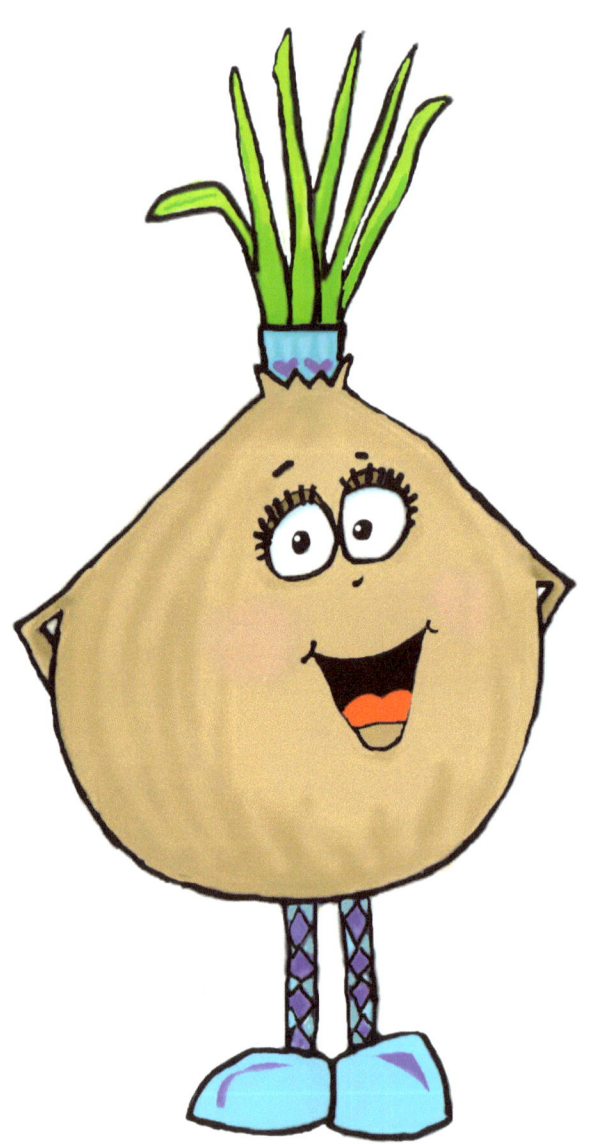

May I introduce... **Mary Onion!**
She makes us laugh till we cry with her funny jokes.

The Amazing Journey of Clarence Carrot

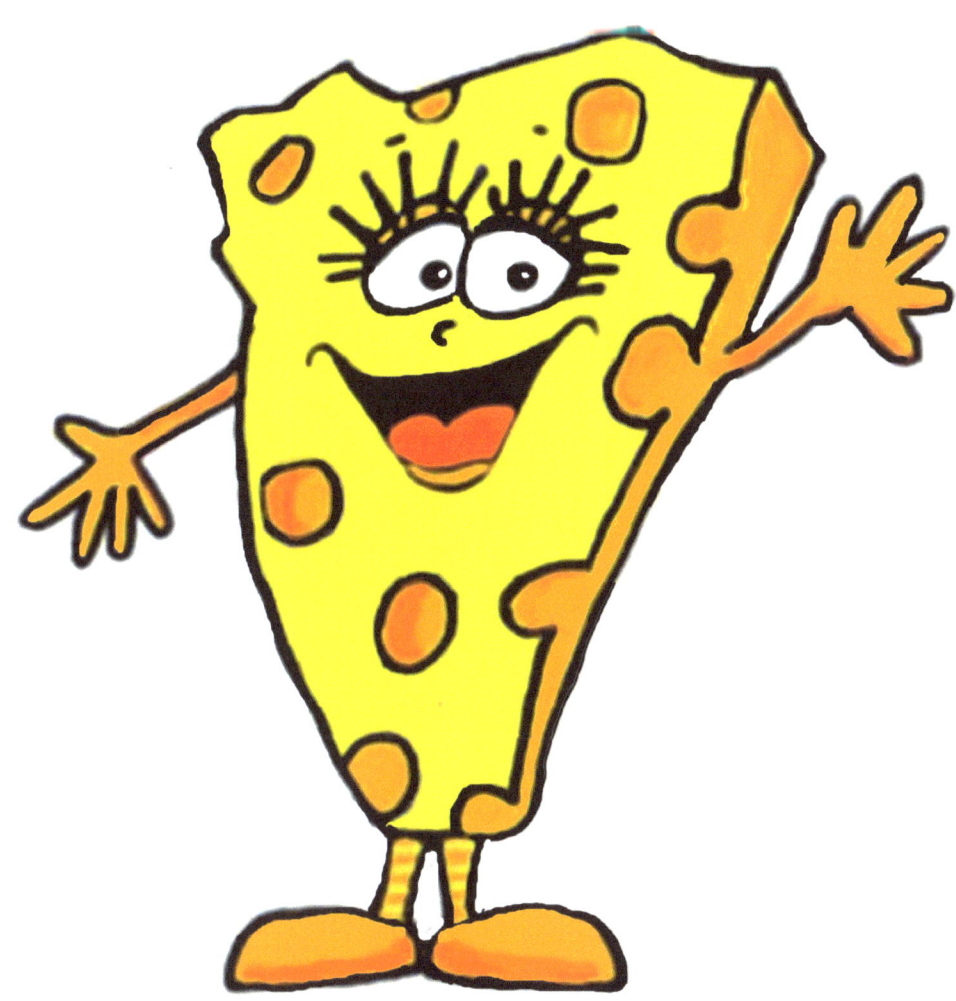

Here comes **Reece Cheese!**
He jumped from his toast, off the breakfast table, to join our group.

The Amazing Journey of Clarence Carrot

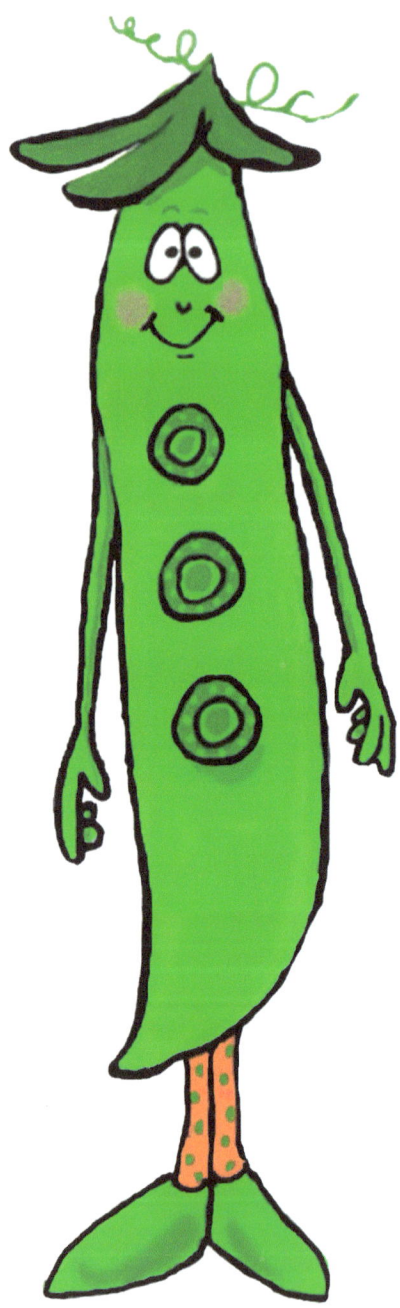

This is **Gene Bean!** His family members come in many shapes and colors and have the funniest names, like: Garbanzo, Navy, Black-Eyed Pea.

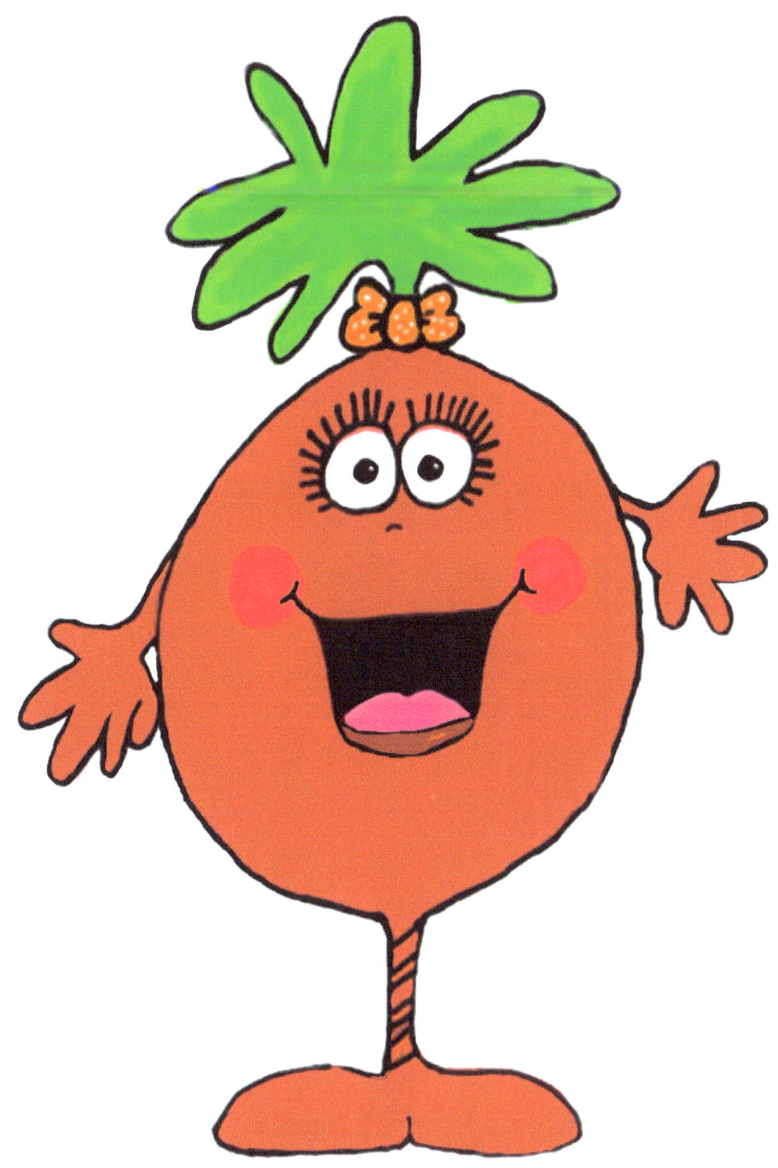

Another good friend... **Trish Radish!**
She is a cute rootlet, but sometimes is a little bit shy.

The Amazing Journey of Clarence Carrot

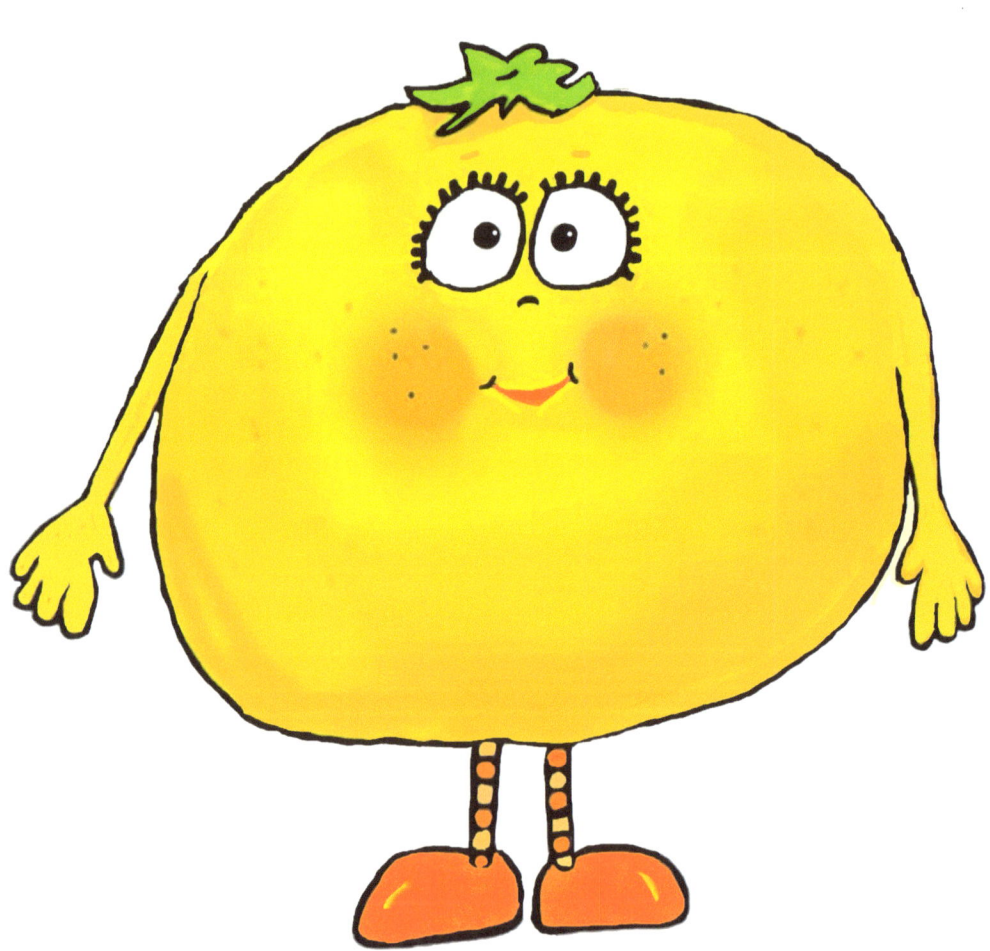

And last but not least, **Ruth Grapefruit!**
She is very curious and loves the sunshine.

Clarence Carrot likes when we call him "Taste Champion" because... he is "Taste Champion"! He will teach you everything about tasting! Do you know how he became "Taste Champion"? Listen...

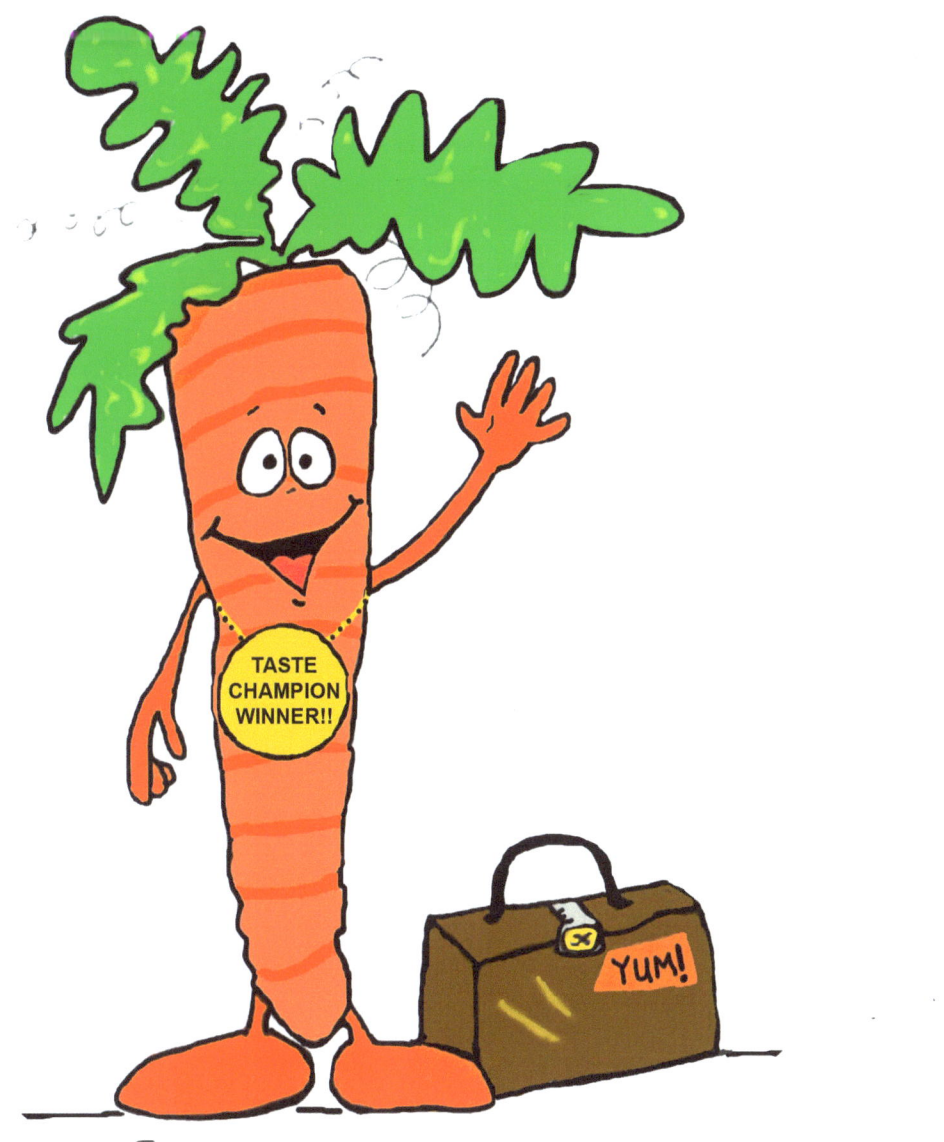

Tom Tomato's Birthday Party

Not too long ago, there was a birthday party for Tom Tomato.

Tom loves to fill his belly, and he almost likes everything. For his party, Mom Tomato organized a big race, a taste race! She placed little plates with bite-size pieces of fruit, vegetables, or other goodies, along the vegetable garden fence.

"Okay," Mom Tomato said, "the eight of you have to line up. I'll explain the game: you taste what is on the first plate, then the second, and so on, until you get to the last plate. The one who tastes the most things will become Taste Champion! When I whistle, GO!"

Round # 1: Apple
On the first plate were pieces of apple. Everybody likes apple so that was easy. They were happy that they all could go to the second plate! Eight tasters were left.

Round # 2: Cheese
The next food to taste was cheese.
"No problem," laughed Reece Cheese. **"I love it!"**
They all clapped their hands.
But Mary Onion started to cry loudly.
"Waaa! Waaa! Waaa!" Big tears rolled over her round cheeks.
"I...I don't like cheese," she sobbed.
She flat-out refused to give it another try. That's why she couldn't go to the next round.
Seven tasters were left.

Round #3: Strawberry
Now they all got a strawberry. Do you know what color a strawberry is?
"That's a beautiful berry!" yelled Tom Tomato. It was okay that he yelled because he was the birthday kid.
"Of course you would say that, Tom; you like all small fruits and veggies!" joked Reece.
Trish Radish started to blush. **"That strawberry looks a little bit...weird!"**
She didn't want to taste, and Bonnie Broccoli also walked away.
"Sorry," Bonnie said, **"but I am still enjoying the cheese, no place for the strawberry yet."**
Five tasters were left.

Round # 4: Banana

Little pieces of banana were on the fourth plate. Gene Bean became a little bit angry.
"I only like red fruit," he said, and he stomped his foot on the ground.
Ruth Grapefruit didn't want to taste either.
"This looks as soft as muddy clay, and that makes me say, NO WAY!" she said and left the race.
"Mmmm, I LOVE Banana; it is sweet and creamy!" laughed Clarence.
Three tasters were left.

Round # 5: Cauliflower

They all 'eyeballed' the next plate. There sat little white florets.
Do you know which vegetable that would be?

"That has to be cauliflower!" shouted Gene Bean cheerfully.
Too bad, he was already out of the race and couldn't taste anymore.
Clarence stuffed his mouth full of the little florets. Reece Cheese couldn't taste anymore.
"This is not for me," he whispered, and he stepped aside.
Too crunchy, way too crunchy!" he mumbled in Gene Bean's ear.
Only two tasters were left.

Round # 6: Lemon

The last round!
It's was Clarence Carrot competing against Tom Tomato.
It was his birthday, should Clarence let him win?
Mom Tomato had put little yellow slices on the last plate.

"I've never tried that," said Clarence to Tom.
"Me neither," answered Tom.

Clarence Carrot knew it was lemon, and his mom once told him that lemons are very sour.
"That's so sour it will twist your tongue into a knot!"
he said to scare Tom Tomato a little bit.
And it worked!

Tom didn't dare to taste it. Clarence took a tiny little nip of the lemon.
Everybody started to laugh. He didn't know why.
"You made such a funny face!" the friends cried!

It was super sour! He thought maybe his tongue should twist into a knot! Clarence Carrot got a big hug from Tom Tomato! All the friends shouted: **"Hurray for Clarence!"** while Mom Tomato clapped her hands and gave him a big medal. That's how Clarence Carrot became "Taste Champion".

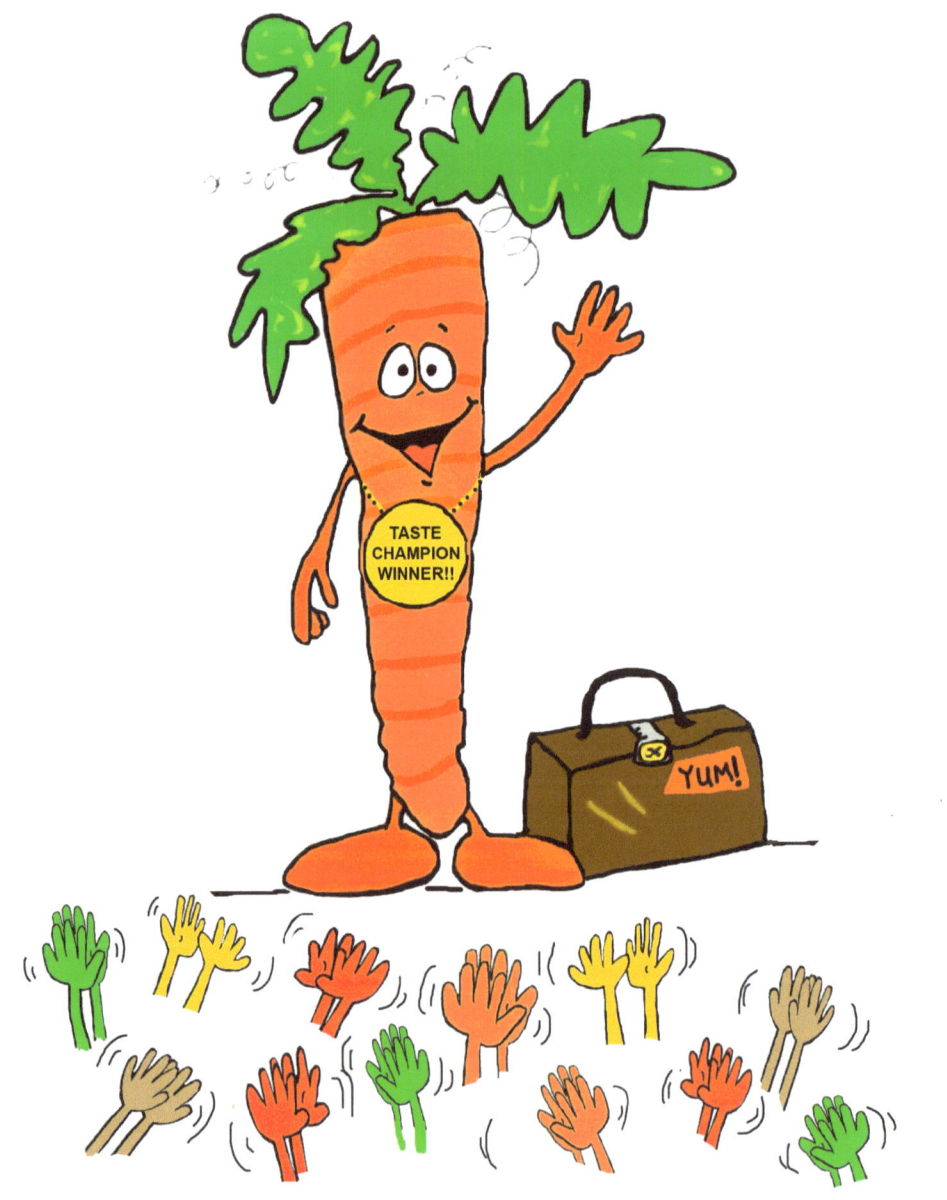

The Amazing Journey of Clarence Carrot

After the birthday party they lay on their backs, looking at the stars and dreaming of distant countries and great adventures. They played 'I spy with my little eye' until they fell asleep.

The next morning the friends heard that the owner of their garden was going to participate in a contest.

"WHO HAS GROWN THE MOST BEAUTIFUL VEGETABLE OR FRUIT IN THE GARDEN?"

They didn't want to end up in a beauty contest,
so they decided to run far, far away and start an Amazing Journey...

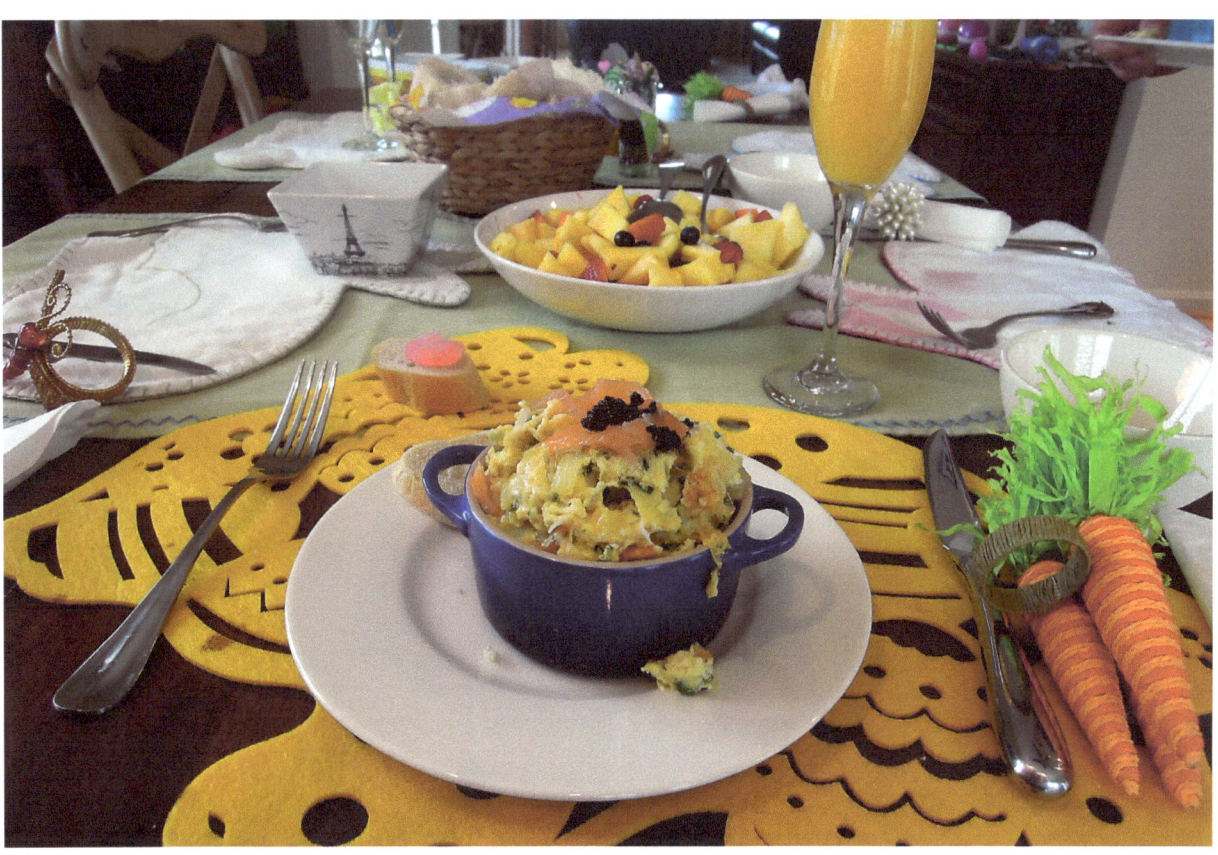

CHAPTER FIVE

Introduce the Five Senses

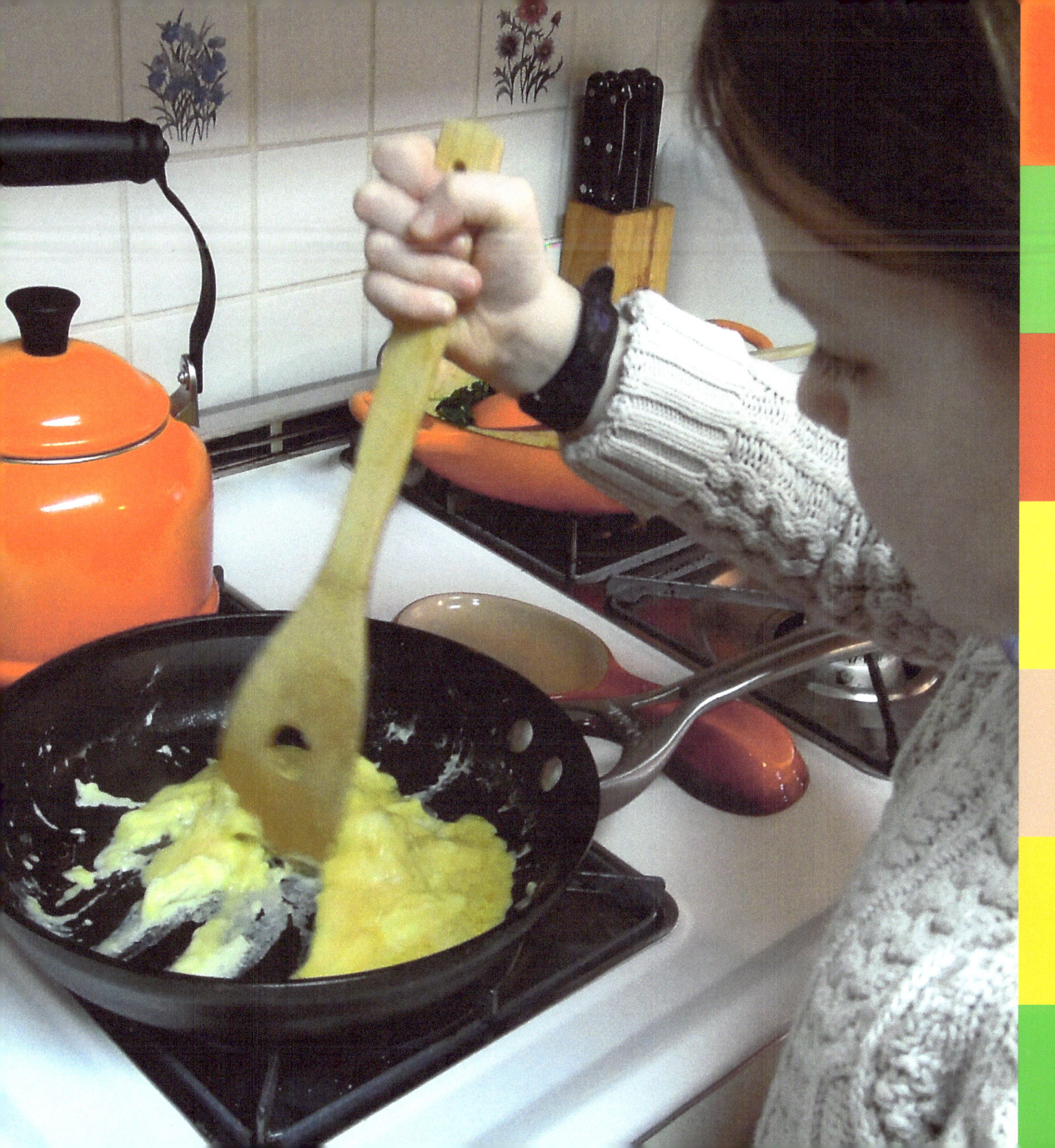

Show the suitcase covered with stickers and let the children 'discover'... the pictograms of the Five Senses.

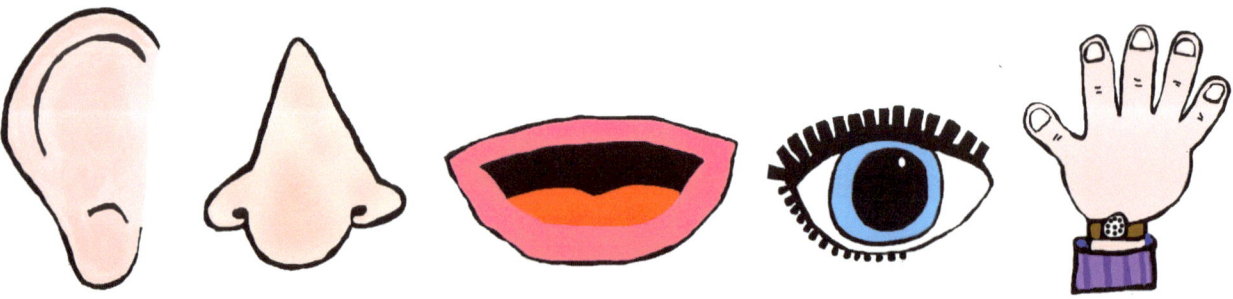

As you talk about the five senses, point out that not everyone has all of them. Children with differing abilities might not be able to see or hear or even smell or taste.

You'll see that many activities incorporate more than one of the senses. Multisensory activities satisfy all learning styles and foster well-rounded, intelligent children.

Open the suitcase, and show the five bags. The children will discover the same pictograms! Each bag represents a different sense and contains the materials needed for the activities featured with each story. (Except fresh foods when asked for.)

Explain to the children that you will tell a different story (each day/week depending on your schedule) and that each bag contains special things for doing fun activities!

Activity 1: A Sensory Stroll

To introduce the theme of the five senses, take the kids on a sensory stroll to the **local produce store**, the **farmers market** or the vegetables and fruits section of the **grocery store**.

Walk around and have the kids examine the world of foods. Ask them what they see. Have them describe what they hear. What kinds of smells are in the store? Find fruits and veggies to taste for the upcoming activities of the program. You can finish the field trip with a picnic and/or a visit to a playground.

If this is logistically impossible, then assign this as an activity with their family! Let the parents know that the children will be discussing their sensory experience at the next class.

Activity 2: Make a Book
Have pictures of what you can find in the store and put them in the book. This will help the kids to remember the ways they use their senses. Print off pictures from your computer before the class or let the children cut out pictures from magazines. Use stapled construction paper.

Activity 3: Who is Who??
Let the children re-tell the story of Tom Tomato's Birthday Party. Use the pictures. Every round you can show the picture of the friend that drops off and of the fruit or vegetable they have to taste. Depending of the children's age you can review parts of the story first as you are passing out the pictures of the friends and also the fruits/veggies.

Questions you can ask before or after:
> What is the name of the 'Taste Champion' ... ?
> How many friends does 'The Taste Champion' ... have?
> Whose birthday party was it?
> Which food did all of the friends like?
> Who was in the last round of the taste race?
> Which food made Clarence have a funny face?

Activity 4: Tasting for Beginners
Re-enact the story with the children and let them taste the apple, cheese, strawberry, banana, cauliflower and lemon. Who is going to taste just like Clarence Carrot???

Tasting and Emotions
Tasting can trigger several emotions. Each child will react differently when he or she does not like a food. Talk with the children about the emotions of different characters in the story. Show a picture, and ask which food the character did/did not want to taste. Also ask about their reactions: angry, sad, shy, happy...
> Everybody likes apple so that was easy. Everybody was ...
> But **Mary Onion** started to cry loudly. She was feeling ...
> **Trish Radish** started to blush. She was feeling a little bit ...
> **Gene Bean** felt .... and stomped his foot on the ground.
> **Ruth Grapefruit** felt ... and said NO WAY!

Encourage the children to talk about their own emotions.

Show the children their 'Taste Pass'.
They will earn stamps/stickers after each activity they complete successfully.

CHAPTER SIX

The Amazing Journey

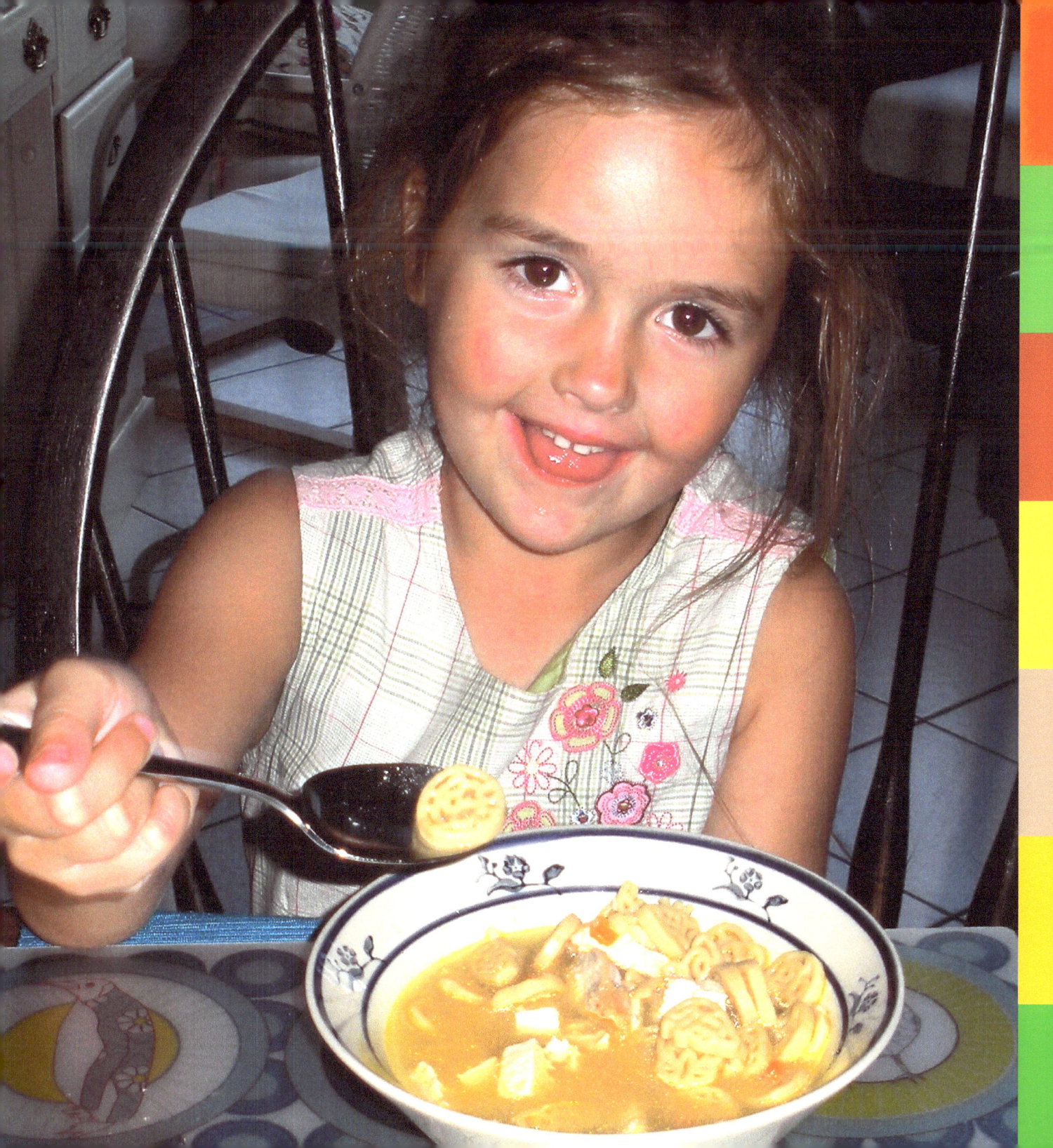

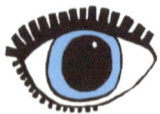

The Amazing Journey of Clarence Carrot

Goals of the Chapter
> Children will enjoy the pictures.
> By asking direct questions, children will develop their powers for keen observation.
> Children will express their observations.
> Children will be able to identify with the pictures.

Time
30-40 minutes

Materials
The **'View Bag'** with 20 different photos of international kids eating or cooking.

Setting
An open space. Children sit in a circle.

Before you start to tell the story, take the 'View Bag' out of the suitcase. Show the pictogram and let the children react freely.

Clarence Carrot and his friends visited gardens, farms, farmers' markets, grocery stores, and the kitchens of all kinds of people. They met new fruit and vegetable friends.

They saw hundreds of things to eat in as many scents and colors, shapes and sizes. Clarence wanted to share these new edible discoveries with you, so he drew and painted them!

He mixed colors: banana-yellow, sea-nymph-blue, crocodile-green, pink-panther- pink, goldfish-orange... He kept his art collection in his travel case. After he painted everything and everyone that he actually saw, he started to paint his dreams.

Have you ever dreamed about fruits and vegetables dancing to the music of a fruity band? He did! There were laughing coconuts and rapping bananas dancing in red skies, and everywhere floated berries and nuts looking at the world with wondering eyes.

And thousands of people: big and small; happy and smiling; having a lovely, cozy time sitting at the dinner table or having a summer picnic in a park.

Sometimes in the night, the wind blew the pictures around and around, high in the sky, until they fell somewhere on a spot where people could come and admire them.

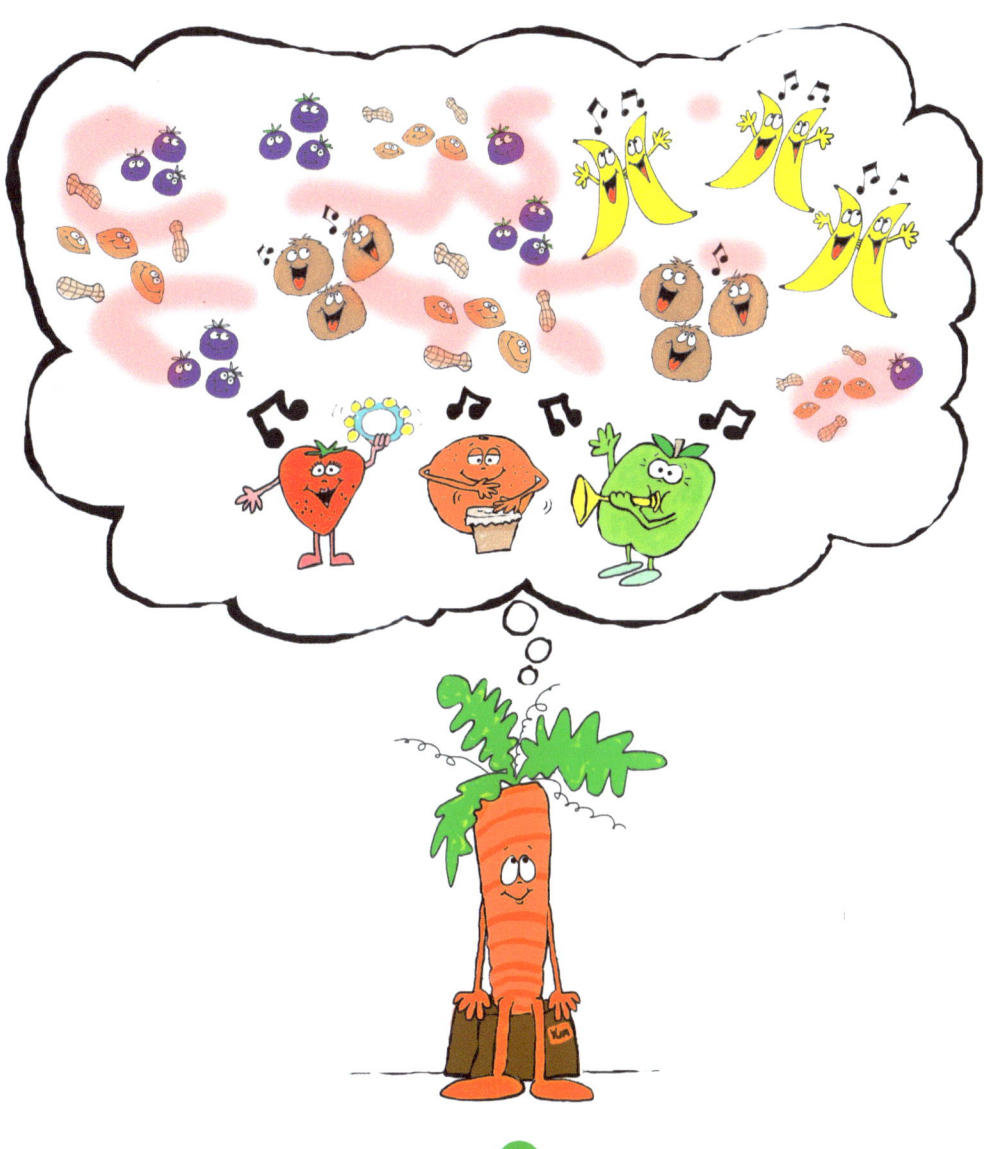

Activity 1: Photo Friend

Material
20 pictures of local and international children eating or preparing food.

Preparation
Play music in an open space. At the end of the story, when you talk about the wind blowing the pictures around, spread the pictures on the ground.

Action
Advise children that they will be selecting a photo "friend." Let the children walk around to look at the pictures. When the music stops, they choose one and sit down.

Observation
Ask specific questions about their favorite photo friend, such as:
> What caught your eye about your friend's photo?
> Why did you find it so special?
> What is your friend doing?
> What is your friend eating? Preparing?
> What is the color of the food?
> Have you ever tasted or eaten that food?
> Look at your photo friend's face.
> Look at his or her eyes, nose, and mouth.

Close your eyes:
> What color are your friend's eyes, hair, clothes?
> Is your friend smiling, angry, sad, or just calm?
> Can you make the same face as your photo friend(s)?

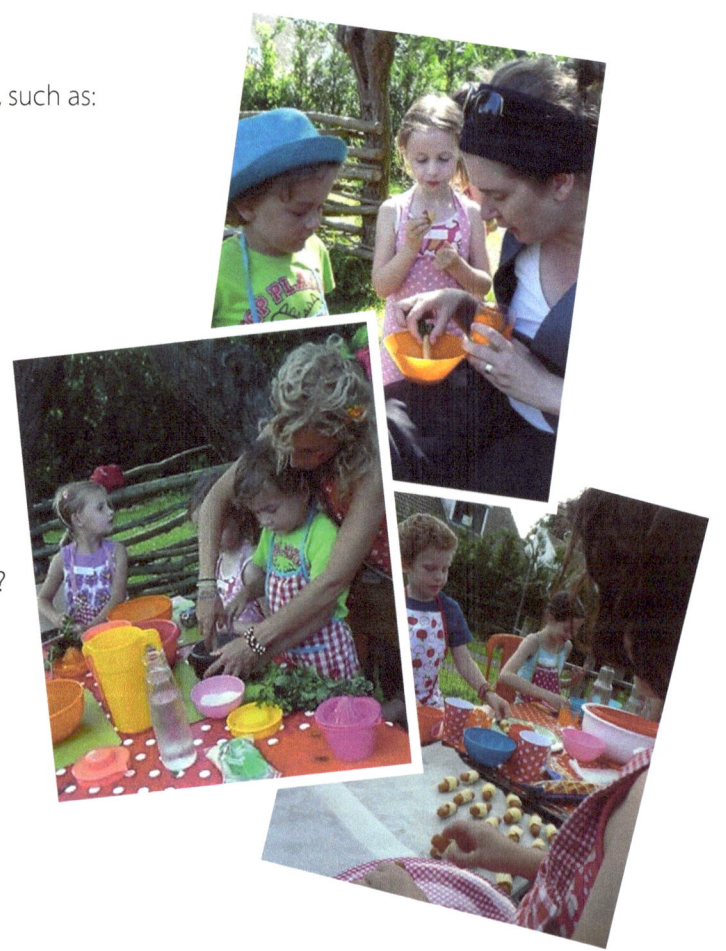

Activity 2: Let's Make a Little 'Elf' Poem
Look at your photo:
> Tell or write something that you see (1 word)
> Describe what you see (2 words)
> Say or write where or when your photo was taken (3 words)
> What is happening? (4 words)
> Surprising end (1 word)
> Altogether, this poem has 11 words. (Eleven is "elf" in Dutch)

Chefs
Two sisters
In the kitchen
Preparing a vegetable soup
Yummy!

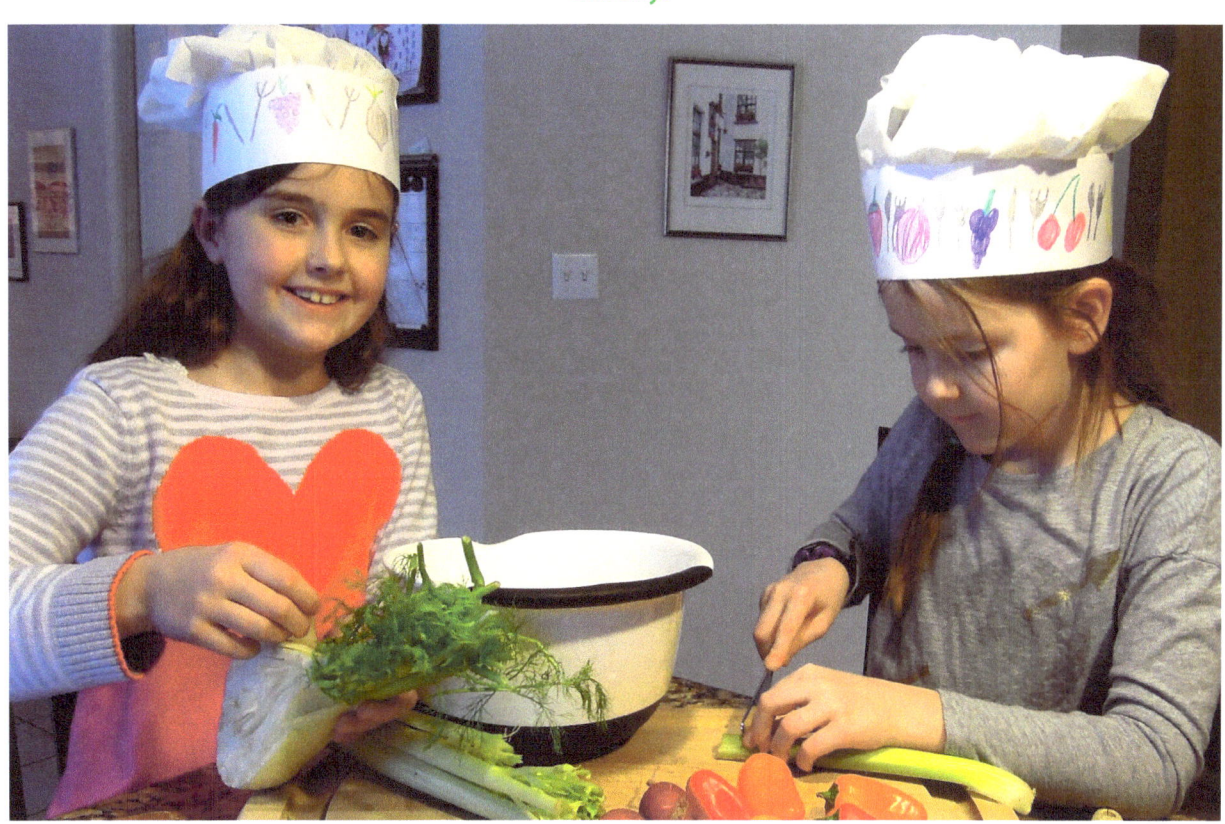

Activity 3: Puzzle Game
Cut pictures into thirds, fourths, or in half. Cut at least three or four pictures. Ask the kids to try to put the pictures back together the right way.

Activity 4: Play Copy Cat
One child thinks of an action related to eating or food. For example: eating an apple or tasting a piece of lemon. Everyone else must watch and then copy it.

Activity 5: Magnifying Glass
Have children observe and describe fruits and vegetables using a magnifying glass. Ask questions like:
> What's the color?
> What's the shape?
> What is the texture - bumpy, smooth, etc.?
> Does it look yummy?

Conclusion:
There is quite a variety of fruits and veggies. Kiwis are very different from bananas or cantaloupes or watermelon or pineapples or blueberries – and veggies are diverse as well.

Activity 6: Traffic Light
Make two cards: one with a red apple (red light or a stop sign) and another with a green apple (green light). Hold up the green light and have the children walk, run, or dance around in a circle.

They need to watch to see when you hold up the "stop" light. When you do, they should stop.

Activity 7: Explore Colors
Encourage kids to find pictures of veggies and fruits in rainbow colors and make a collage or another arts and craft project.

Feel free to add more visual acitvities. Be creatieve and have fun!

The Amazing Journey of Clarence Carrot

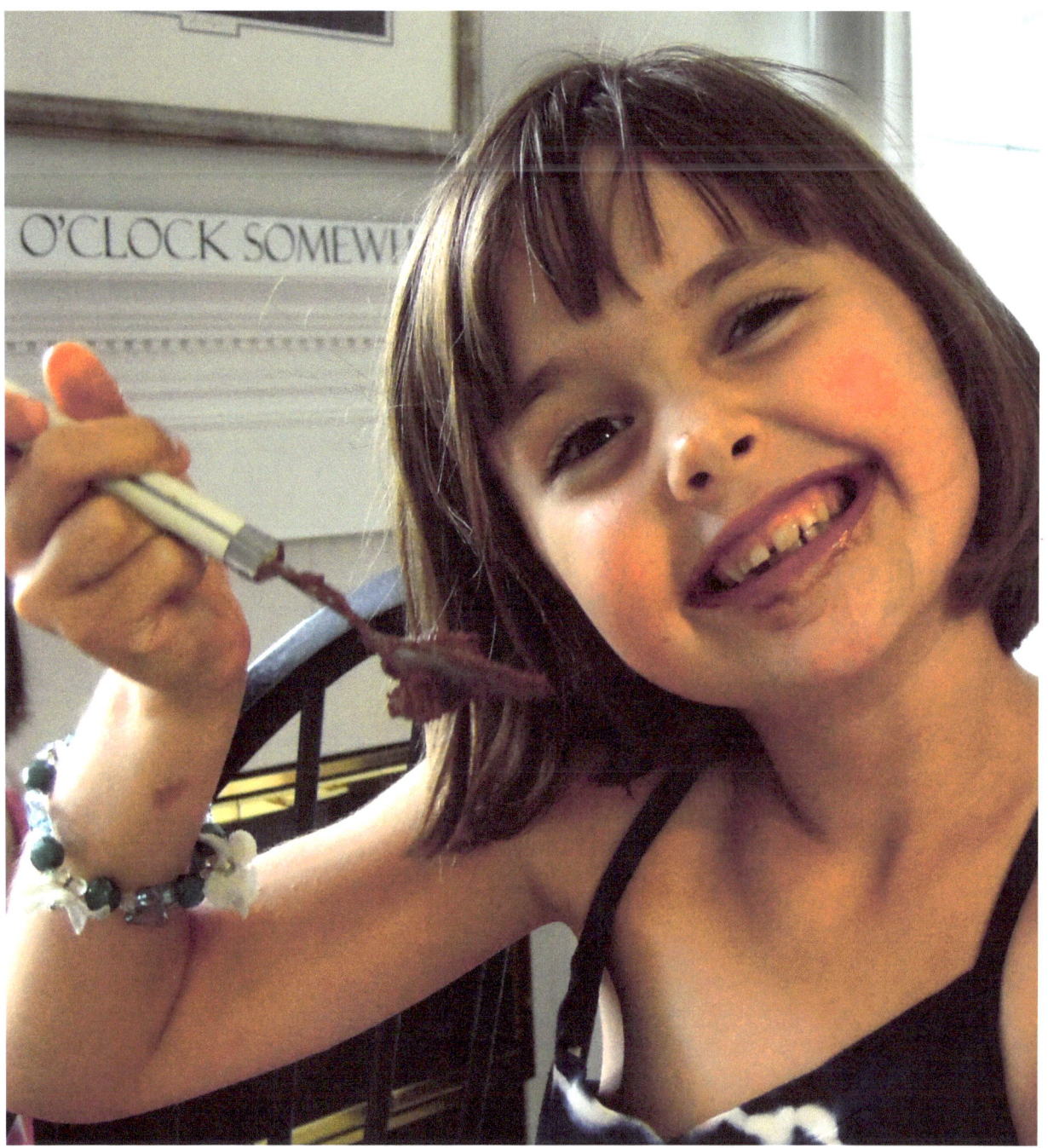

CHAPTER SEVEN

The Little Honey Bread

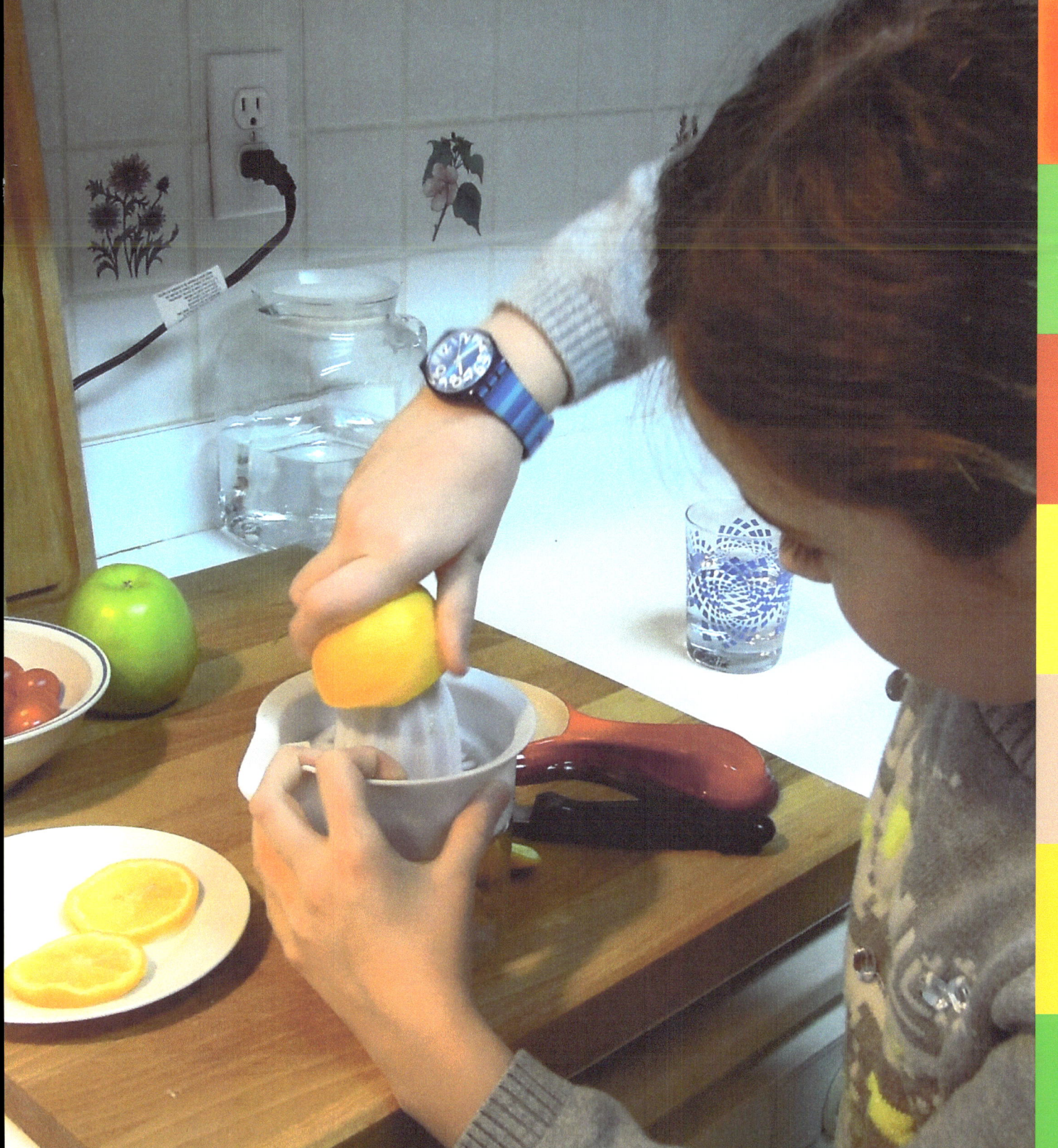

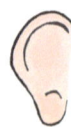

> ## Goals of the Chapter
> > Children will be stimulated to express themselves, with special attention to rhythm.
> > Children will create music with "strange" instruments.
> > Children will develop their attention span by listening and focusing on the different parts of the story.
> > Children will listen to the "food song."
> > Children will discover that pleasant background music can help them to feel relaxed.
> > Children will use words like crunchy, cracker, crispy...
>
> ## Time
> 30-40 minutes
>
> ## Materials
> > Illustrations
> > Instruments
> > Music CD
>
> ## Setting
> An open space. Children sit in a circle.

One morning when Clarence Carrot woke up, a smell was tickling his nose. He sniffed and inhaled deeply.

"Hmmm." Clarence was curious.
"What is smelling so sweet and cozy? I've GOT to find that delicious smelling thing!"

He walked in the direction of a little house near the edge of the forest. The smell became more and more intense, the closer he got to the house. Clarence looked through the open window and there it was! On the kitchen table was a little bread, warm and smelling like honey and cinnamon.

It was a little Honey Bread! Clarence Carrot stepped closer to see it with his little eyes and to smell it with his nose. He was just about to touch the bread, when it opened one eye and then the other, and a big smile came on its face.

All at once, Honey Bread popped off the table, jumped out of the window, and rolled till it scooted over the fence! It rolled and rolled and rolled, further into the forest. Suddenly a big hare hopped out of the bushes!

"Hello, Little Honey Bread, you look so yummy... I'd like to taste you!"
"No no, Long Ear, that's not possible! But I can sing a song for you."

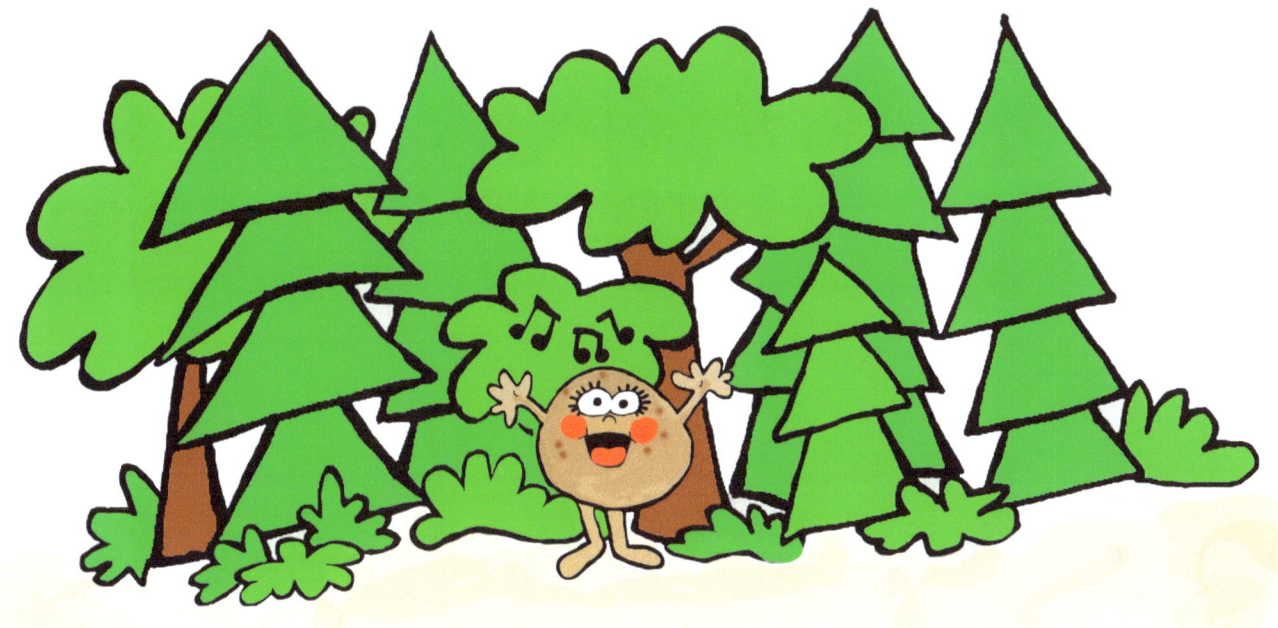

Bread is a lovely thing to eat.
Honey Bread is a special treat.

Patted and rolled,
Shaped and baked.
From many tasters I've escaped.
I'm smart and I'm free.

You cannot catch me.
Before you try,
I'll say bye bye!"

Little Honey Bread rolled further away through the forest. Then a wolf saw the cheerful little bread.

"Hello, Honey Bread, you look so yummy... I'd like to taste you!"
"No no, Mr. Grey Wolf, that's not possible! But I can sing a song for you."

> Bread is a lovely thing to eat.
> Honey Bread is a special treat.
>
> Patted and rolled,
> Shaped and baked.
> From many tasters I've escaped.
> I'm smart and I'm free.
>
> You cannot catch me.
> Before you try,
> I'll say bye bye!"

Again, Little Honey Bread rolled further away until it met a hungry Bear.

"Hello, Little Honey Bread, you look so yummy... I'd like to taste you!"
"No no, Grumbling Bear, that's not possible! But I can sing a song for you."

> Bread is a lovely thing to eat.
> Honey Bread is a special treat.
>
> Patted and rolled,
> Shaped and baked.
> From many tasters I've escaped.
> I'm smart and I'm free.
>
> You cannot catch me.
> Before you try,
> I'll say bye bye!"

Little Honey Bread rolled further and further and met the smart Mr. Fox.

"Hi, Little Honey Bread, you look so pretty and cheerful today."
After those flattering words, Little Honey Bread lay down, relaxed, and sang its song.

>Bread is a lovely thing to eat.
>Honey Bread is a special treat.
>
>Patted and rolled,
>Shaped and baked.
>From many tasters I've escaped.
>I'm smart and I'm free.
>
>You cannot catch me.
>Before you try,
>I'll say bye bye!"

Little Honey Bread wanted to continue its walk in the forest, but smart Mr. Fox said, **"Oh, what a lovely song! So sorry that I didn't hear it very well. I am a bit deaf. "** Come and sit on my snout, closer to my ear, and sing the song another time!"

Little Honey Bread jumped on the sharp snout of smart Mr. Fox and started to sing its tricky song.

>Bread is a lovely thing to eat.
>Honey Bread is a special treat.
>
>Patted and rolled,
>Shaped and baked.
>From many tasters I've escaped.
>I'm smart and I'm free.
>
>You cannot catch me.
>Before you try,
>I'll … …

The Amazing Journey of Clarence Carrot

And when the song was almost finished, the smart fox jerked back his head, caught Little Honey Bread and ate it all up.

Note
I got this story of The Little Honey Bread from my Bulgarian friend Elena Alexandrova. She got it from her mom, who got it from her mom, etc...

Let the children react freely if they recognize the story-line of the 1875 story, The Gingerbread Man. Folktales of the runaway food type are found in Germany, the British Isles, and Eastern Europe, as well as in the United States.

Reflection
What do you think of the story? Was it funny? Exciting? Surprising? Encourage the children to share freely.

Activity 1: Explore the Instruments
Pass out the instruments and let the children experiment for a while. Talk about the instruments and explain where they come from and what they are made of.
> What do they sound like?
> Are they difficult to play?
> Does your instrument look like an instrument you know?

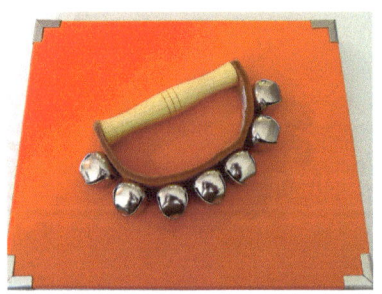
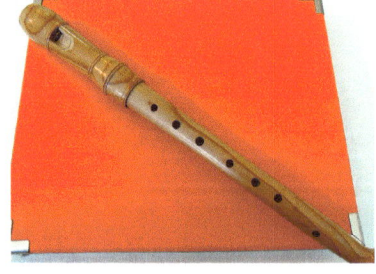
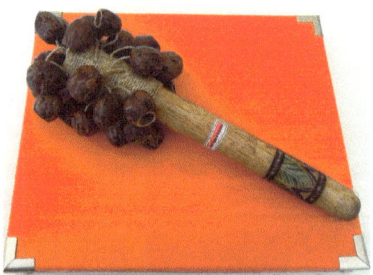
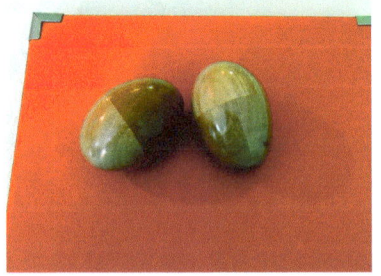
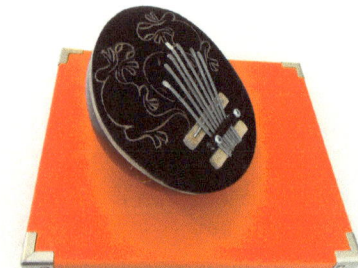
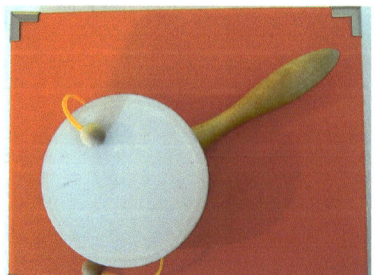

Activity 2: Tell the Honey Bread Story Again
Every child will use their instrument and have a role to play in the story.
- **Clarence Carrot**: the calabash shaker
- **Little Honey Bread**: the ankle bells
- **The hare**: the bean bag
- **The wolf**: the fruit rind shaker
- **The bear**: the coconut thumb piano
- **The fox**: the flute

Let the children use the instruments during the Little Honey Bread song!

Activity 3: Move and Play
Go outside, on the playground, in the gym class...
Let the children act out the story, with and without the instruments.

Activity 4: Bake and Taste
Here is a simple bread recipe with a twist - the addition of honey. You will be surprised how simple it is to make this delicious Honey Bread. Baking bread is such a fun activity to do with kids. Measuring, scooping, and kneading provide wonderful sensory and fine motor opportunities! Besides, who can resist the smell!!

When scheduling this activity, note that the bread will take about an hour to rise, and another 1/2 hour to rise after being kneaded, plus 30-35 minutes to bake.

You will need:
- 1 package of active dry yeast
- 1 1/4 cup of warm milk (110 to 115 degrees)
- 1/4 cup of honey
- 1/8 cup of melted butter
- 1 teaspoon of salt
- 4 cups of all purpose flour
- Small piece of foil

Dissolve one package of yeast into a bowl of the warmed milk.
Next add the honey, melted butter, and salt.
Mix to combine.

Add 3 cups of flour (slowly, a bit at a time), and mix with hands until a soft dough forms.
Save the last cup of flour for dusting and kneading.

Place the dough on a floured surface and knead for about 10 minutes.
This is the favorite part for kids. They love punching, pulling, and squeezing the dough.

When you are done kneading, place the dough in a greased bowl and cover it.
Place the bowl in a warm place so it can rise and double in size. This will take about an hour.

Next, punch down the dough, and place it in a greased loaf pan.
Cover the dough and place in a warm place for another 30 minutes until it rises and doubles again.

After 15 minutes into the second rise, pre-heat the oven to 375 F.
Bake for 30-35 minutes.

When the top starts to brown, at about 20 minutes, place foil over the pan for the remainder of the cooking time. Remove from pan when done, and allow it to cool off before tasting.

Enjoy the Honey Bread!

Activity 5: Snaps, Crackles, Pops, and Crunches

Serve rice crispies for snack. As you pour the milk over the cereal, let the children listen to the cereal and talk to them about snap, crackle, and pop.

Serve a carrot, an apple, or a celery stalk (let the children choose). Have them listen while they take a bite. Talk to them about crunch.

Note
Try the healthier brown rice breakfast cereal puffs.

Conclusion
The things we eat make different sound

Activity 6: Listen and Dance to the Song

Put a Little Sunshine in Your Mouth

It's amazing how a little sunshine
Some dirt and water and a little time
Grow fruits and vegetables of every kind
Put a little sunshine in your mouth
Chase those tired blues away
You only need five servings a day
You'll have more energy to run and play
Put a little sunshine in your mouth

chorus:
Put a little sunshine in your mouth
'Cause bein' healthy's what it's all about
It'll make your whole body wanna scream and shout
Put a little sunshine in your mouth
Put a little sunshine in your mouth
'Cause bein' healthy's what it's all about
It'll make your whole body wanna scream and shout
Put a little sunshine in your mouth
Put a little sunshine in your mouth

Just take that ripe banana peel
Pull it down and make a meal
You won't believe how good you'll feel
Put a little sunshine in your mouth
Put some veggies in your hand
Very soon you'll feel grand
Your heart will beat like a marching band
Put a little sunshine in your mouth

chorus
If you want to shine like a superstar
It makes no difference just who you are
Fruits and vegetables will take you far
Put a little sunshine in your mouth
Just sitting still is such a bore
So what on earth are you waiting for
Your health is knocking at the door
Put a little sunshine in your mouth

Words & Music by James B. Coffey, M.Ed.
Performed by James B. Coffey

**Let the children put a stamp in their Taste Pass
and congratulate them for the great listening job!**

CHAPTER EIGHT

Fun at the Farm

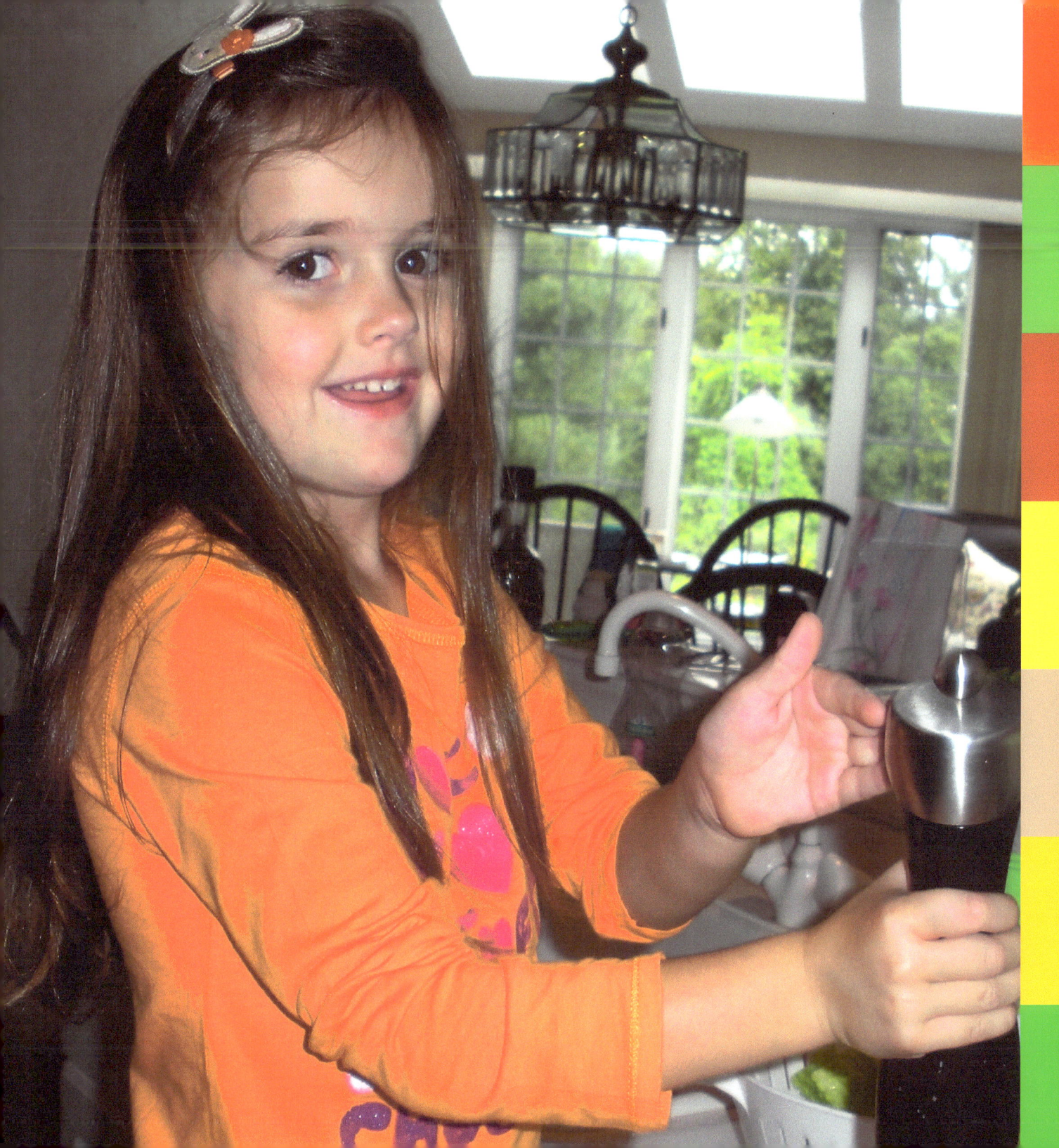

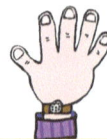

Goals of the Chapter
> Children will understand why the apples and pears choose a walnut for playing soccer.
> Children will be challenged to play soccer.
> Children will experience shapes and textures of fruits and vegetables.
> Children will describe fruits and vegetables by shape, color, size, or other characteristics.
> **"Resistance"** for tasting will disappear.

Time
30-40 minutes

Materials
> Pictures of the different characters
> Touch Box
> Apple, pear, walnut, pumpkin and other vegetables and fruits and their pictures
> Template for a chef's hat

Setting
Children sit in a circle or in a group.

It was a cool, autumn night. Clouds floated in the dark sky. Farmer Joe and his family were fast asleep in the farm house. They had worked all day picking apples and pears in the orchard. The big baskets sat overflowing in the barn, filling the air with a fresh fruit smell.

It was calm and peaceful when Clarence Carrot and his friends entered the dark barn. Suddenly the moon emerged from behind a cloud and shone through the window. The whole barn lit up.

They heard footsteps and there was Dustin Pumpkin with a whistle between his lips and a brown walnut in his hands.

"Let the soccer game begin!!" he shouted, and he whistled three times.

FWEET... FWEET... FWEET!!!

A team of apples climbed down from one basket, a team of pears from another. Dustin Pumpkin whistled again and threw the walnut in the air. The apples and the pears did all they could to kick the walnut into the goal.

"This is hilarious!" said Clarence the Carrot to one of his friends. The whole barn echoed with shouts of cheering fruits and veggies!

At the end of the game the score was 3 for the apples and 2 for the pears. **"That was fun!"** everybody exclaimed. **"We challenge you to a rematch, and next time we will win!"** shouted the pears. And before the moon disappeared and the sun woke up, the barn became quiet and peaceful once more.

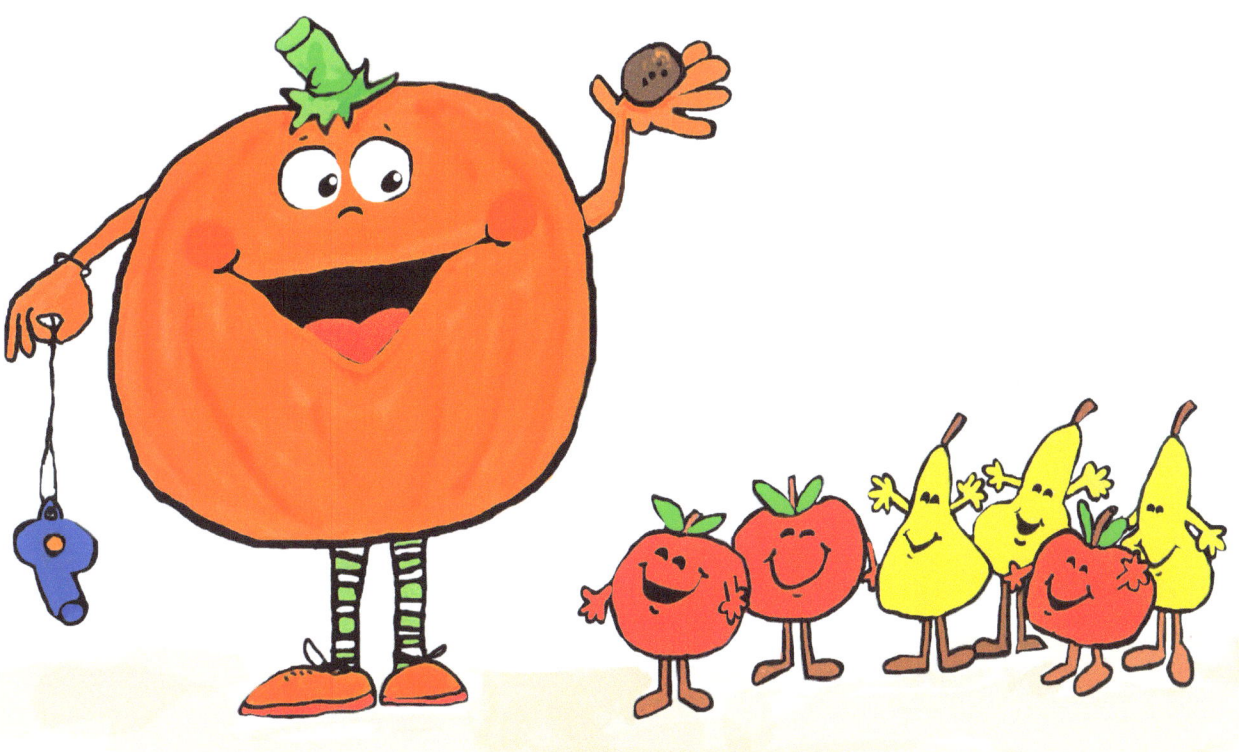

Reflection:
What do you think of the story? Was it funny? Exciting? Surprising? Let the children share freely
Let them touch the real stuff (apple, pear, pumpkin, walnut), and have kids place them on the pictures of the characters in the story. Encourage them to describe the produce by shape, texture, peel, skin...

Ask questions:
What kind of "ball" did the fruits use for playing soccer? Can you explain why?
Name other vegetables or fruits that have a round shape. Could they use them for playing soccer? Explain.

The Touch Box

You will need fruits and veggies with different shapes and textures. Be aware that several little hands will touch the produce. It is advised not to put a tomato or berries in the Touch Box.

Take care that the children stay in front of the Touch Box so they cannot peek. You can put a napkin or towel over the box to avoid that temptation.

Activity 1: Search for the Carrot
Place a carrot in the Touch Box in advance. Let them touch what is in the box. After they each take a turn, ask them to guess what is in the box.

Activity 2: Choose and Touch
Let one of the children put something in the Touch Box. Meanwhile, have the other children close their eyes. Let the children touch and guess. Let each child take a turn to put a fruit or veggie in the box.

Activity 3: Guess What I'm Feeling
While the children watch you, put several pieces of produce in the Touch Box. Select one child to choose something in the Touch Box. The others have to guess which fruit or veggie their friend is touching. Without naming it, the child describes what it feels like.

For example, for a cucumber: it is long and slender; it has a green skin; when you take a bite, it is crunchy and moist; you can slice it into circles; and it is tasty in a salad. You can ask questions of each child like: Is it big or small? Is it soft or hard, bumpy or smooth? Does it prick or stick?

Activity 4: Little Chefs

To make a chef's hat, you need: a soft tape measure, a piece of white card, a ruler, a pencil, scissors, white crepe paper or a white paper tablecloth about 30cm x 60cm, sticky tape

Step 1: Measure all the way around the child's head over the ears using a soft tape measure. Then measure and cut out a strip of card an inch longer than the length you measured and about 5 inches high.
Step 2: Now fold the strip of card in half LONGWAYS then unfold it.
Step 3: Lay one of the long edges of your crepe paper or tablecloth on top of the card so it meets the fold of the card. Stick one corner of the paper to the card.
Step 4: Make about 10 little folds along the same edge of the paper to gather it up. Stick them to the card as you go along.
Step 5: Fold up the bottom edge of the card then bend the two ends of the card to meet each other. Overlap them slightly then stick some pieces of tape all the way up the join.
Step 6: Gather up the top of the paper to make a point and wrap some sticky tape around it.
Step 7: Push down the point inside the hat then pull it down from the inside, making the hat puff out.

Decorate and let the children enjoy wearing their chef's hat!

Activity 5: Chop, Slice and TASTE!

Use the produce that the children have touched. Rinse the fruits or veggies that have no peel; let the children wash their hands. Explain that a knife can be dangerous, and have them watch you use it safely. Let the children arrange the slices and pieces on plates and little by little they will become "little Chefs"!

Let the children put a stamp in their Taste Pass and congratulate them for the great touch job!

CHAPTER NINE

Mia Bella and the Little Cloud

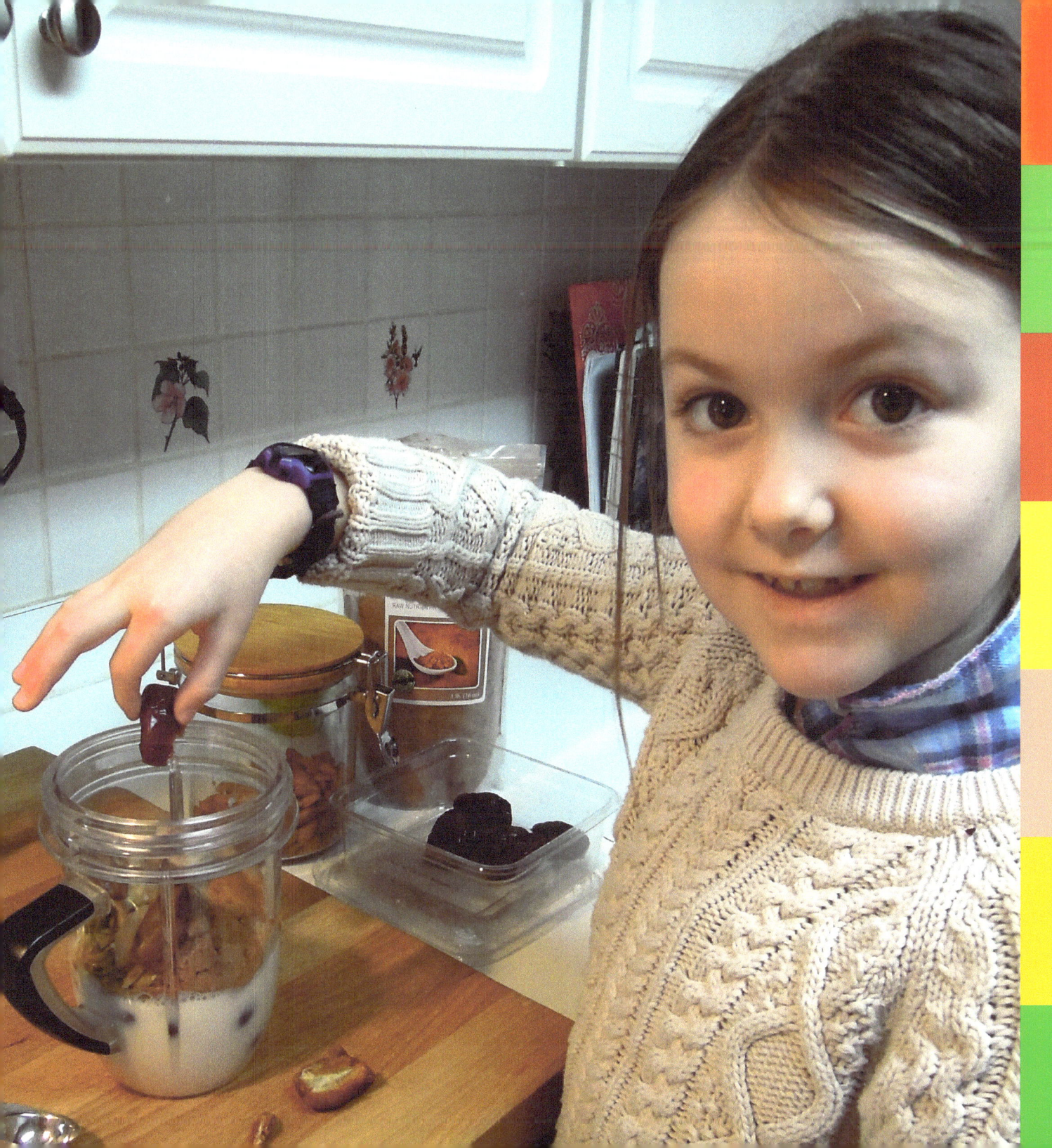

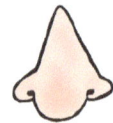

Goals of the Chapter
> Children will recognize different smells.
> Children will experience how smell impacts taste.
> Children will associate smells with different environments and surroundings.
> Children will develop their attention span by listening and focusing on the different parts of the story.

Time
30-40 minutes

Materials
> Pictures of the different characters
> The Nose Knows Matching Game
> Smell boxes with 6 different pieces of veggies or fruits

Setting
Children sit in a circle or in a group.

In a country, far away from here, where it is always summertime, there was a tiny, little cloud. His name was Claudio. He floated, all by himself, in the clear, blue sky. If you listened carefully, you could hear him sobbing softly, and if you looked closely, you could see tiny drops sprinkling down from the little cloud.

Mia Bella, the rainbow bird, had taken off on her early morning flight. Still sleepy, her eyes were not open yet. Boink!!!! She crashed against the little cloud!

"Look out!!" she squawked. **"The sky is not all yours!!"**
"Oh! Pardon, but I cannot see...," said Claudio. "**I was floating with my mommy and daddy and grandma and grandpa and the whole family, but I've lost them...**"

Mia Bella's anger disappeared. She felt so sorry for the child cloud. The rainbow bird thought deep, deep thoughts in her bird head.

"**Maybe I can help!**" she said. "**I will fly ahead and look for your cloud family. When I find them, I will send them back to you!**"

Claudio started to brighten.

"**Fly fast and come back soon! I hope you will find them!**" he said. Mia Bella stretched her colorful wings, shook her little head, took a deep breath, and set off to fly over the wide world.

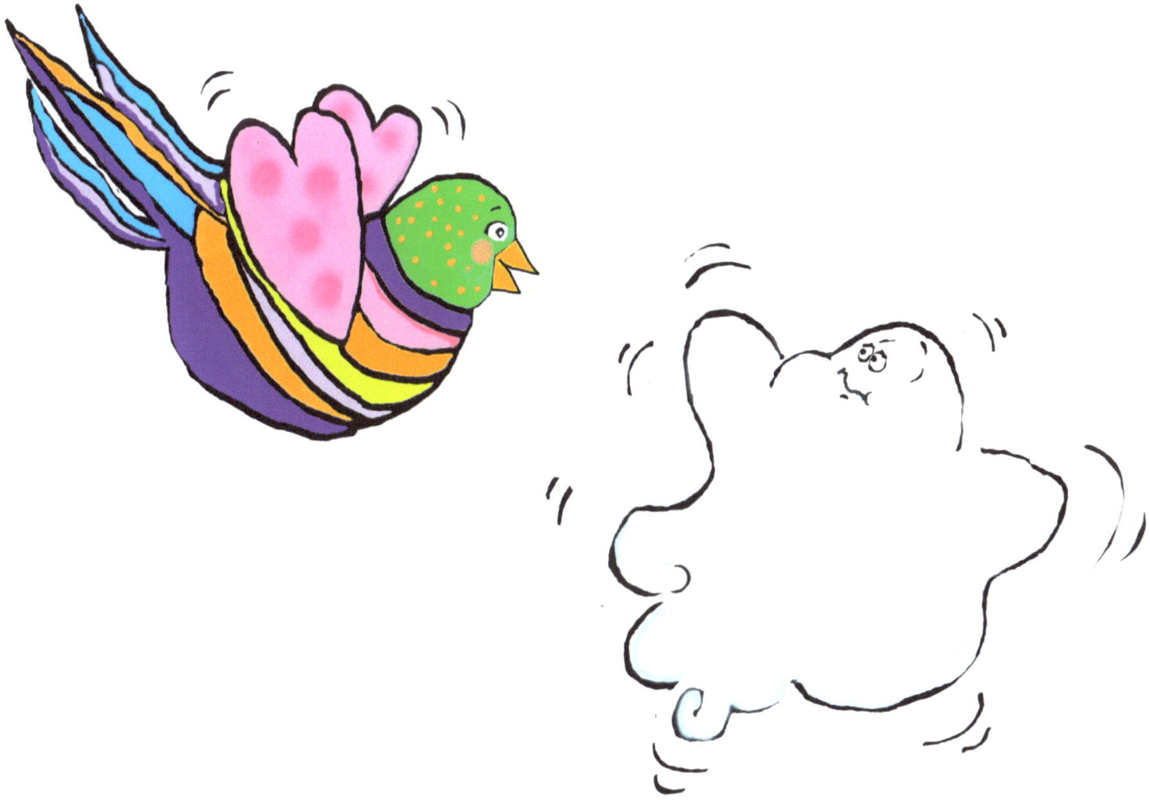

First she whooshed over the ocean. Then over the countryside, where she glimpsed people having a party. Further on, she flew over green fields. She flew farther and farther over highways. When she was almost on the other side of the world she finally found Claudio's family.

The cloud family looked heartbroken - grey and heavy. They dropped big tears down to the earth.
Mia Bella tweeted loudly to get their attention.

"Hi there!! Your cloud child, Claudio, is looking for you! Come and join me! I'll take you to him."

But the clouds were too heavy. They could not follow Mia Bella. Again the rainbow bird thought deep, deep thoughts in her bird head.

"No problem," she said, "I will fly back by myself and bring Claudio to you!"

Mia Bella stretched her wings, shook her tail, and returned - over the highways, over the big green fields, over the countryside where people were enjoying their party, and over the big ocean. She flew against the wind, flapping her wings. "Flap, flap, flap." Completely exhausted, she finally met up with Claudio.

"Did you find my family?" asked the little cloud, worried.
"Yes! Yes! Far away from here," whistled Mia Bella, almost out of breath.
"They were too heavy with sorrow at your disappearance to follow me."
"How wonderful that you found them! Yay! I want to see them! Now! Now!" said Claudio.
"Will you show me the way?"

"I want to," said Mia Bella, "but I am so tired. I would like to sleep for 100 nights. I can barely lift my wings, and they are on the other side of the world." Now Claudio started to think deep, deep thoughts in his cloud head.

"Tell me how to find my family. I will go by myself!"
"But you cannot see," sighed Mia Bella.
"I can smell and touch and taste and hear! Tell me the things you remember!"

The rainbow bird started to describe her long journey.

"Well, first, you will fly over the ocean. It will smell a little salty, a bit fishy, and you will hear the water making a roaring noise and sometimes the breeze blows ferociously stormy.

After that, you will float over the countryside. The air will smell delicious from the aromas of roasted onions; carrots; salmon and beef; warm baked bread; fresh, green salad leaves and tomatoes; olive oil; and herbs. You will hear happy people laughing and children singing and playing.

They are having a party. Then you will hear the leaves on the trees rustling; you'll smell the rich, earthy moistness of the crops growing in the fields.

**Further on, you will sniff a yucky smell coming from cars.
You will hear: Honk! Honk! Vroom! Vroom! And it feels a little bit... smoky-grey.**

Mia Bella almost fell asleep.

"OK!" said Claudio. **"I will float as fast as I can to my family!
Thank you so much, my friend. Thank you for your help, Mia Bella."**

Mia Bella did not hear Claudio's happy words. She had fallen fast asleep on top of the downy cloud. Softly they floated in the sky. After the trip to the other side of the world, Mia Bella suddenly woke up.

What a funny feeling! At first all she saw around her was white.
Then she realized she was in the middle of the snuggly, puffy hugs Claudio was receiving from his family.

Reflection
What do you think of the story? Was it funny? Exciting? Surprising? Let the children share freely.

Sense of Smell
The sense of smell is probably the most disregarded sense, but it is more important than most of us realize. Food would taste bland if we couldn't smell. Think about when you have a stuffy nose. Does food taste different? Scent also attracts us to beautiful things like flowers and repels us from germy things like trash.

Activity 1: Tasting Without Smelling
Get some nose plugs or nose clips. (If you can't find them, the children can pinch their nostrils closed like when they dunk under water.) Let the children eat bites of food with and without their noses smelling. Do the foods taste different?

Everything has a particular scent. Think about how the foods you love smell. Scent is linked with memory. So smelling certain things can make you feel happy because you remember somebody important or a special time.

Activity 2: The Nose Knows Matching Game
Smelling scents in bottles provides a wonderful learning experience for kids. It helps develop their senses and encourages them to use more than just their eyes when solving problems. These activities challenge children to identify smells, sort scents, and match smells.

The smell game has two equal sets of 6 bottles containing different scents (put some cacao, thyme, lemon, mint, coffee, vinegar, cinnamon or vanilla, almond,... extract on a cotton ball).

Let the children test each bottle. Then instruct them to place the matching bottles, two-by two

Reflection
> Was it hard to find the matching smells?
> What smells did you know?
> What smell did you like the most?
> Which one did you not like?

Activity 3: Smell Boxes

Fill the smell boxes (tin or plastic containers with holes punched in the lids) with 6 different, small pieces of veggies or fruits. Do not peel, as this will help the food aromas last.

Choices may include: onion, orange, mandarin, lemon, banana, celery, red bell pepper, etc. It is helpful for young kids to see the open boxes before they do the smell test.

Show pictures of each fruit or vegetable.

Pass the smell boxes to the children.
Let them take a whiff and decide which fruit or veggie is in the smell box.

Instruct them to put their smell box with the matching picture.

Open the smell boxes so the children can see what they have smelled.

Conclusion
Everything we eat has a specific smell.

Let the children put a stamp in their Taste Pass and congratulate them for the great smell job!

CHAPTER TEN

Meeting Sisters Sweet, Salty, Sour, and Bitter

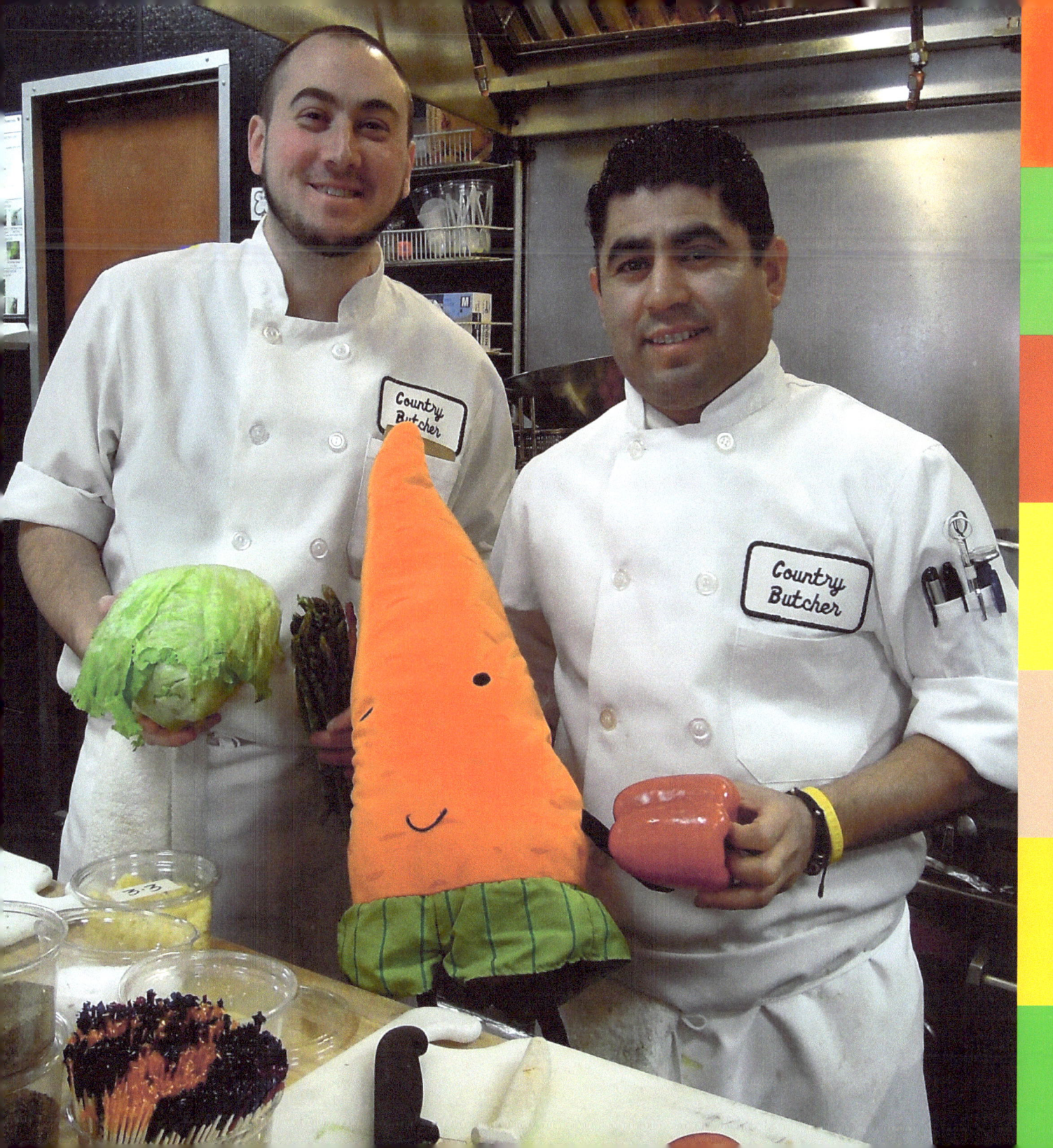

The Amazing Journey of Clarence Carrot

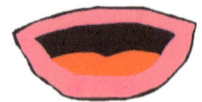

Goals of the Chapter
> Children will recognize and name different tastes: sweet, salty, sour, and bitter.
> They will develop an open mind to learn and accept new tastes.
> Children will focus on different sensorial triggers and get inspired to taste new things.
> They will see their own expressions in the mirror while tasting.

Time
30-40 minutes

Materials
> Pictures of the different taste sisters
> Trays, bowls, and cups in 4 colors: orange=sweet, blue=salty, purple=sour, green=bitter
> Magnifying glasses
> 3 pieces of food for each taste and picture

Setting
Children sit in a circle or in a group.

One day, Clarence Carrot woke up after a nap and felt a little hunger in his belly. He took a walk on Pleasant Street and passed by the restaurant of his great friend, Chef Ollie. The door was wide open. Clarence popped inside; nobody was around.

He walked to the kitchen, calling: **"Chef Ollie! Chef Ollie! Chef Ooooooooollie!!"**
Nobody answered.

Clarence saw four bowls on the countertop filled with food. Now he felt even more hunger in his tummy. Clarence moved in for a closer view with his pointy eyes. In the first bowl he saw a piece of fruit. It was white with a red peel. It smelled fresh and inviting. Clarence smiled.

"I should take a taste," Clarence thought, and he took a bite. "Yummy, crunchy and sweet." He took another bite and another. Suddenly, the bowl moved! Clarence Carrot felt frightened and wanted to run away, but a smiling face appeared in the bottom of the bowl.

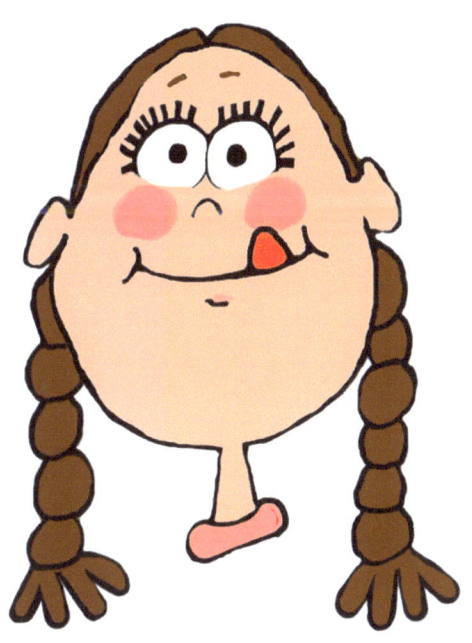

"Hello, Mr. Carrot! I am Sister Sweet!"

"Hi, Sister Sweet; I am Clarence. Nice to meet you! Actually, I'm looking for Chef Ollie. I am a little bit hungry, and I saw that piece of… of…"

"It was a piece of apple, the sweetest apple in the whole wide world!" said Sister Sweet. "My sisters have other tastes; you should try them too! Today is the Taste Festival in Chef Ollie's Restaurant, and he's doing errands in the village."

At that moment Chef Ollie entered his kitchen with bags full of fruits and veggies and cheeses and sausages and much more.

"Hi Clarence," he said, "Welcome to my kitchen!"

The chef noticed the empty bowl.
Sister Sweet whispered in Chef Ollie's ear.

"Clarence, you should taste all the things on the table because you are Taste Champion!" said the chef. Clarence eagerly tried the second bowl, filled with little sticks covered with white crystals.

"These sticks are not sweet; they are crunchy and salty!!" he said. At once, a funny face showed up in the bottom of that bowl.

"Hello, Mr. Carrot! I am Sister Salty!"

"Hi, Sister Salty; I am Clarence. Nice to meet you too!"
"Chef Ollie sometimes adds little bits of salt to make his food more flavorful," said Sister Salty.
"The little white sparkles on the pretzels are salt crystals."

"Good to know," said Clarence, "good to know."

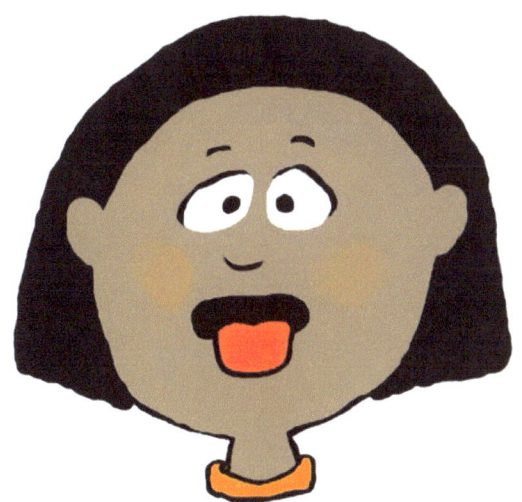

In the next bowl was a piece of fruit that Clarence knew very well!

He had become Taste Champion because of the little yellow wedges. While he licked the lemon wedge, another funny face showed up.

"Hi, Mr. Carrot; I am Sister Sour!"
"Hi, Sister Sour, I am Clarence. Nice to meet you too!"

"Come and look in the mirror while you taste that lemon, then you will see that we look alike!"

And while Clarence tasted the sour juice, he made a funny face. They all laughed.

There was one bowl left. Clarence was not sure if he should try the dark brown pieces in the purple bowl. Carefully, he took a bite.

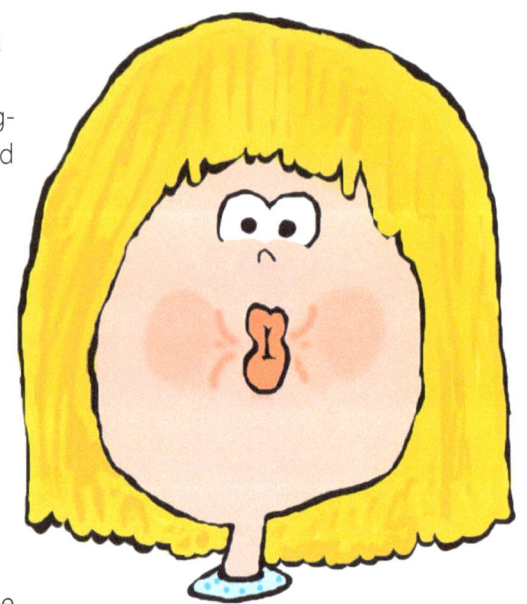

The piece cracked and tasted strange in his mouth.

"Don't worry, Mr. Carrot, I am Sister Bitter!" said the face in the bowl that Clarence had come to expect.
"I am the taste of that piece of bittersweet chocolate!"

"Hi, Sister Bitter, I am Clarence. Nice to meet you!" said Clarence, trying to hide his face. He thought that he was probably making a face like Sister Bitter.

Chef Ollie joined the group. **"Well done, my friend, you are a great Taste Champion,"** said Chef Ollie, clapping his hands. **"I am so proud of you!"**

The sisters cheered. **Bravo!! Bravo!! Bravo!!** "I have a great idea," Chef Ollie said. **"Would you like to help us organize the Taste Festival?** There are so many things to do. You can invite your friends too."

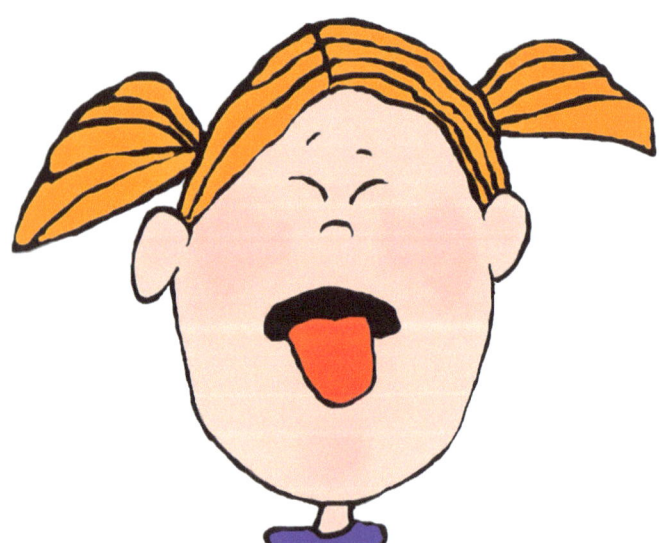

"Sure! Of course! I am happy to help. I will be back with my friends!!" It was an unforgettable festival with the Sisters Sweet, Salty, Sour, Bitter, and lots of friends. Helping Chef Ollie was like a dream come true.

Below are activities to help young children become aware of and have opportunities to sample varieties of taste.

Activity 1: Identify the Four Basic Tastes: Sweet, Salty, Sour, and Bitter
Provide bowls and cups in 4 colors: **orange** = sweet, **blue** = salty, **purple** = sour, **green** = bitter
Fill the twelve containers with:
> Sugar, pieces of mint candy, honey, banana
> Lemon wedges, pickles, plain yogurt, green apple
> Salt, salted pretzels, parmesan cheese, salted water
> Unsweetened baker's chocolate, radish, grapefruit, celery tops

Place the containers on a table. Give the children "taste" plates/cups and a small spoon/tooth pick. Give them also glasses of water to cleanse their palates.

Let the children explore the plates and bowls using a magnifying glass. Let them share their observations.

Ask questions like:
> What is the color?
> What is the shape?
> Does it look yummy?

Conclusion
All foods look different.

Taste the sugar. This is **SWEET!**

Taste the salt. This is **SALTY!**

Taste the lemon. This is **SOUR!**

Taste the baker's chocolate. This is **BITTER!**

Activity 2: Can You Recognize Sweet, Salty, Sour, and Bitter in a Variety of Foods?

Taste each of the other foods, and decide which of the above four tastes it is most like.

Place the foods with similar tastes with the matching pictures. You will probably come up with four groups of three foods each: three sweet things, three salty, three sour and three bitter. If not, that's okay! The important thing is to explore the sense of taste. All flavors are made up of some combination of these tastes.

Explain to the children that when we taste, we also use our other senses. Things that look yummy make us curious to try them. Give the children time to observe each food before tasting. Let them try closing their eyes before sampling, which can be a bit strange. Let the children watch themselves in a mirror while they taste. Can you see on people's faces if they like it or not? Sometimes when we taste something sour or bitter, we make funny faces.

Ask children after each tasting whether they liked it or not. Compare the different reactions. If they don't want to taste some of the foods, you can encourage them by letting them watch themselves in the mirror and have fun with the silly expressions on their faces.

Make the children feel comfortable and let them share freely.

Conclusion
We have our own preferences.

Activity 3: Salted Water

Give each child a little straw, and let them taste some water. Let them react freely.

Then, let them taste lightly salted water. Allow them to react freely.

You can let them taste highly salted water too.

Conclusion
Sometimes things can be very salty, and sometimes things can be a little bit salty. People can make things more salty by adding salt. Explain to children that adding too much salt can change the real taste of foods and can make foods taste yucky.

Activity 4: SWEET Tooth

Ask children what they think about the sweet samples. Let them name more examples of sweet tasting foods: banana, cookies, candy, apple juice, etc.

Ask them which foods are healthier, and which foods are less healthy. Do they know the difference? Which foods help their bodies grow healthy and strong?

Ask children how often they eat cake. Ask them how often they eat apples. Cakes are for parties, and apples you can eat everyday!

Conclusion

Our bodies will be healthiest if we eat lots of fruits and vegetables everyday and save cookies and candy for special occasions!

Let the children put a stamp in their Taste Pass after each tasting and congratulate them for the great taste job!

CHAPTER ELEVEN

Finale: An Unforgettable Taste Festival

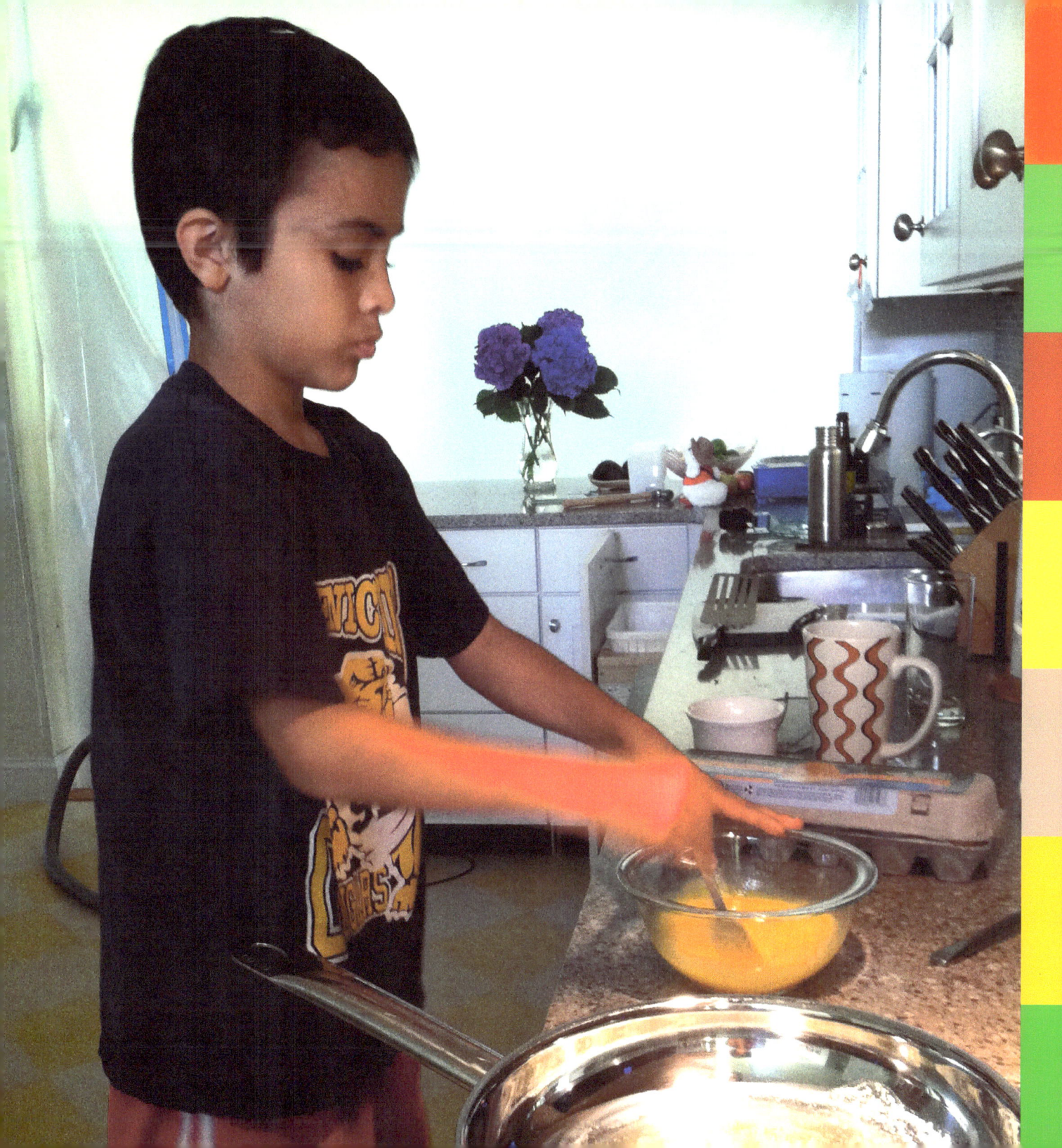

To celebrate this Amazing journey of tasting new foods, it's time for a Taste Festival.

The guest of honor is "Clarence Carrot" and all his friends are coming. The suitcase is ready, and Clarence will have a great meal before he leaves for another Amazing Journey. For these activities you can invite parents and work with volunteers!! Use your creativity and enjoy!!!

Activity 1: A Fruity Atmosphere
Decorate the room with pictures and crafts

Activity 2: A Medal for the "Taste Champions"
Reflect with the children about their taste experiences. Did they taste new foods? Did they enjoy the activities? Let the children color and decorate their medal, using pencils, paint, beans, lentils, etc.

Glue the medal on a piece of cardboard; staple a nice ribbon on it.
Organize an official moment with music and big applause.

Activity 3: Young Chefs
> Prepare and enjoy a healthy meal or snack with the children.
> Advise them to wash their hands before starting.
> Give good guidance about the foods and the tools.
> Use terms like "spread butter or cheese with a knife," "scoop little pieces of fruit and veggies with a spoon."
> Use a fork or a wooden pick for tomatoes or berries.
> Let the children touch the foods. That will make them confident related to the texture and more eager to taste.
> Let them decorate their own (whole wheat) sandwich with lots of veggies, such as shredded carrot, sliced tomato, cucumber, lettuce, radish, red beet...
> Make nice plates with fruits or fruit skewers for dessert.

Activity 4: Cheers!
Serve "healthy" drinks like water, iced mint tea with honey, milk, fresh juices, smoothies…

Activity 5: Let's Move!
Invite the children outdoors on the playground or indoors in a gym class. Choose some volunteers. They will be the "blenders." The other children are the fruits. The blenders need the fruits for making smoothies. The fruits don't want to fall into the hands of the blenders. The blenders have to touch the fruit children. When a fruit child is touched, they have to take your hand. Be sure you are in the middle!

The captured fruit children make a line by holding each other's hand. When a free fruit child touches the line, the captured fruit children are free again. The blenders have to protect the line and try to touch fruit children. The blenders have won when all the fruit children are captured.

Activity 6: Dance to the Music!
Play the **"Fruit and Veggie Song"** and let the children move freely.

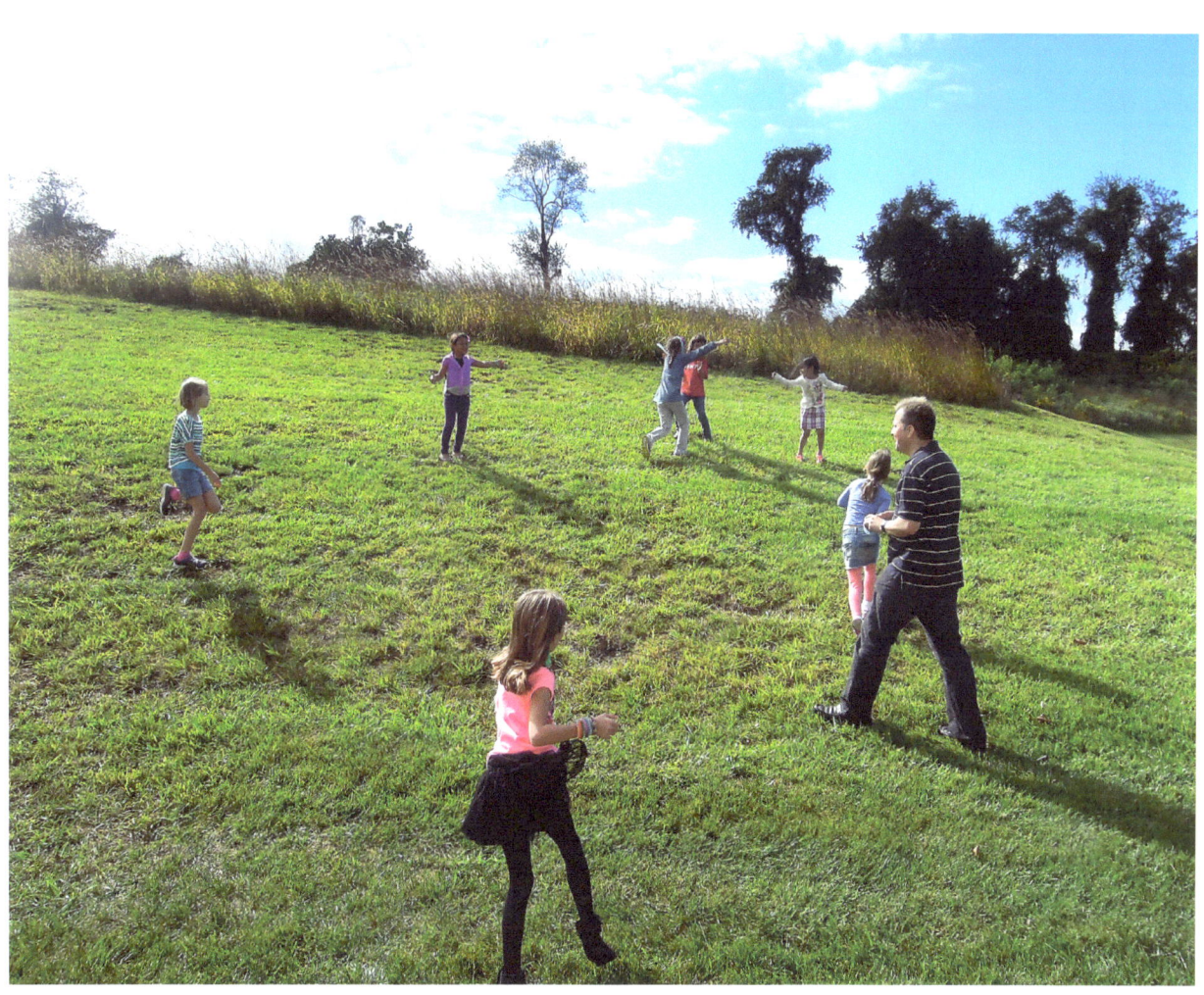

THE SUITCASE

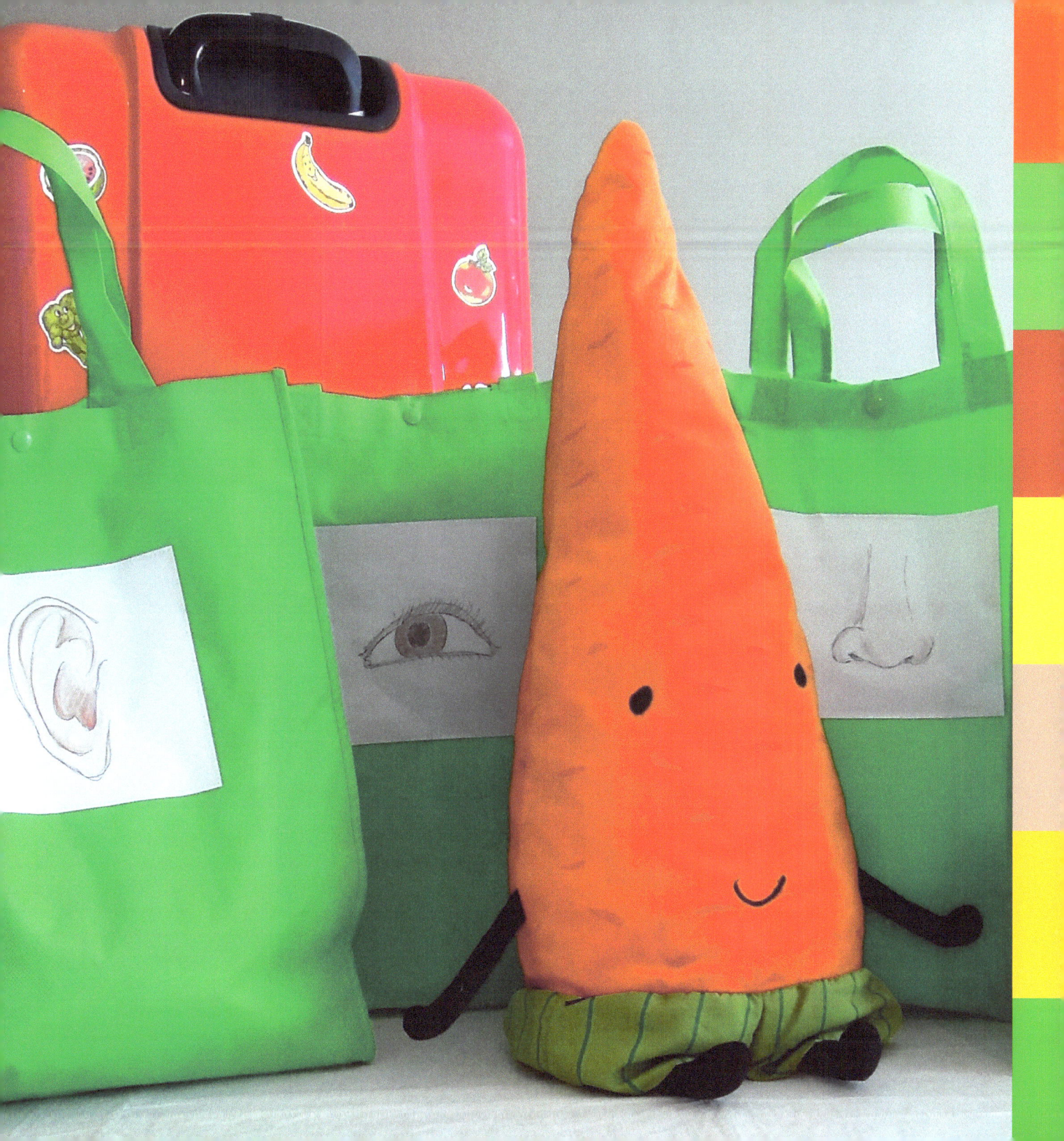

All Materials Needed for the Program

- A big suitcase with the 5 senses bags
- Clarence Carrot in a basket
- Pictures of the 8 characters
- Pictures of an apple, cheese, a strawberry, a banana, cauliflower and a lemon
- A Taste Pass for every child
- Stamps or stickers

5 bags with all the material belonging to each story/sense:

The 'View Bag'
- 20 different photos of kids eating or cooking
- Puzzle Game
- Magnifying Glasses
- Traffic Light: two cards: one with a red apple and one with a green apple

The 'Hear Bag'
- Pictures of the Little Honey Bread story
- Instruments
- Ingredients for baking
- Ingredients for hearing Snaps, Crackles, Pops and Crunches
- Put A Little Sunshine in Your Mouth

The 'Touch bag'
- Pictures of Fun in the Barn
- Apple, pear, walnut, pumpkin or squash...
- Touch Box
- Chef's Hat materials
- Ingredients for Chop, Slice and TASTE!

The 'Smell Bag'
- Pictures of Mia Bella and the little Cloud
- Nose plugs
- The Nose Knows Matching Game: two sets of 6 bottles/jars/tins. Each set contains: 6 different smells. 6 different scents
- Smell Jars for 6 different pieces of veggies or fruits

The 'Taste' Bag
- Pictures of Sweet, Sour, Salty and Bitter
- Trays, bowls and cups in 4 colors:
  orange=sweet
  blue=salt
  purple=sour
  green=bitter
- 3 pieces of food for each taste + pictures
- Mirror

For More information: www.chris4health.com

The Taste Pass

From:

Draw your picture in the middle and place your stickers all around

Acknowledgements

Thank you to the following individuals; without their contributions and support, this book would not have been written:

Joshua Rosenthal and **Lindsey Smith** from the Institute for Integrative Nutrition for their expertise and encouragement throughout this project.
Tracy Hart, my editor, for her expertise and time in polishing my manuscript.
LouLou Clayton, my illustrator, for the lovely illustrations.
Romain Verbeke, my book designer and webmaster, for his original and creative work.
Noah Zingarelli, my buddy, for giving me Mia Bella.
Denise Brown, for the inspiring phone calls.
Bonita Kehler and **Jill Borin** for helping me to "Americanize" my project.
Kathi Hopkins, for proof reading.
Carol Nees, **Lindsey Shaffer**, **Kathi Wellnitzk**, and **Lisa Cypressi**, for encouraging feedback.
My dear friend **Linda Beukelaers**, for helping with Clarence's Suitcase.
The Produce Place in Kennett Square for the nice pictures.
The Country Butcher in Kennett Square for the supportive crew and nice photo of the chefs.
My family and friends, nearby and far away, who contributed to my well-being and happiness in the past and will do so in the future.
My children, **Sam** and **Liesbeth**, for making me the happiest mom in the world.
My granddaughters: **Sophie**, **Molly**, and **Paulien**, for being my never-ending source of inspiration.
My late father in-law, **Frank Mahoney**, for all the support he gave me to pursue my dream.
My husband **Dennis Mahoney**, for believing in me!

Resources

Websites
- www.superhealthykids.com is an online resource for parents who are looking for ideas, recipes and tips for feeding their kids healthier and living better.
- www.choosemyplate.gov
- www.ikea.com
- www.amazon.com

Books

My Snack Size Skills,... 8 life lessons for a healthy Me!
by Janelle Buchheit and Lindsey Smith

In just minutes a day kids can learn powerful life lessons to help them grow into happy and healthy adults that will impact the world in a positive way.

Just Be
by Patricia Bean

This book is written to appeal to toddlers, who will love its simplicity and repetition. However, the book contains ageless wisdom for all readers.

The book reminds the reader to slow down, take a breath, and Just Be! Just Be was illustrated by the author,... granddaughters using handmade paper to create the collage. The colors of the collages in the book correspond to the colors of the rainbow and to the Chakra colors.

Prince Peter Eats the Sun
by Kimmell J. Proctor

Prince Peter Eats the Sun is a foodie fairy tale to enchant all ages. Follow the Prince on his royal journey as he solves the mystery of what it means to eat the sun. This fresh and fun picture book offers food conscious families a kid-friendly, rare resource about the power of eating well. Includes suggested recipes for families to eat the sun at home!

www.ingramcontent.com/pod-product-compliance
Lightning Source LLC
Chambersburg PA
CBHW042139290426
44110CB00002B/56